# Institutional care
# and rehabilitation

Geoff Shepherd

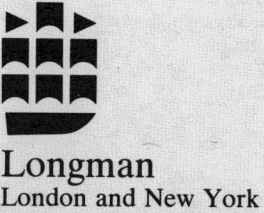

**Longman**
London and New York

**Longman Group Limited**
Longman House, Burnt Mill, Harlow
Essex CM20 2JE, England
*Associated companies throughout the world*

*Published in the United States of America
by Longman Inc., New York*

© Longman Group Limited 1984

First published 1984   496\93097

**British Library Cataloguing in Publication Data**
Shepherd, Geoffrey, 19--
    Institutional care and rehabilitation. –
    (Longman applied psychology)
    1. Mentally ill – Care and treatment – Great Britain
    I. Title
    362.2'1'0941    RC439

ISBN 0-582-29604-8

**Library of Congress Cataloging in Publication Data**
Shepherd, Geoffrey.
    Institutional care and rehabilitation.

    (Longman applied psychology)
    Includes bibliographical references and index.
    1. Mentally ill – Rehabilitation. 2. Mentally ill –
Institutional care. 3. Psychiatric hospital care.
4. Chronically ill – Rehabilitation. 5. Chronically ill –
Institutional care. I. Title. II. Series. [DNLM: 1. Mental
disorders – Therapy. 2. Hospitals, Psychiatric –
Organization and administration. 3. Community mental
health services – Organization and administration.
4. Rehabilitation. WM 400 S548i]
RC439.5.S48    1984    362.2'1    83-12011

ISBN 0-582-29604-8

Set in 9½/11pt Linotron 202 Times
Printed in Hong Kong by
Astros Printing Ltd.

# Contents

To Douglas

# Editor's preface

In most areas of applied psychology there is no shortage of hardback textbooks many hundreds of pages in length. They give a broad coverage of the total field but rarely in sufficient detail in any one topic area for undergraduates, particularly honours students. This is even more true for trainees and professionals in such areas as clinical psychology.

The Longman Applied Psychology series consists of authoritative short books each concerned with a specific aspect of applied psychology. The brief given to the authors of this series was to describe the current state of knowledge in the area, how that knowledge is applied to the solution of practical problems and what new developments of real-life relevance may be expected in the near future. The twelve books which have been commissioned so far are concerned mainly with clinical psychology, defined very broadly. Topics range from gambling to ageing and from the chemical control of behaviour to social factors in mental illness.

The books go into sufficient depth for the needs of students at all levels and professionals yet remain well within the grasp of the interested general reader. A number of groups will find their educational and professional needs or their personal interests met by this series: professional psychologists and those in training (clinical, educational, occupational, etc.); psychology undergraduates; undergraduate students in other disciplines which include aspects of applied psychology (e.g. social administration, sociology, management, and particularly medicine); professionals and trainee professionals in fields outside psychology, but which draw on applications of psychology (doctors of all kinds, particularly psychiatrists and general practitioners, social workers, nurses, particularly psychiatric nurses, counsellors – such as school, vocational and marital – and personnel managers).

Finally, members of the general public who have been introduced to a particular topic by the increasing number of well-informed and well-presented newspaper articles and television programmes will be able to follow it up and pursue it in more depth.

Philip Feldman

# Acknowledgements

It is customary to suggest that far more people deserve a
mention for their contribution to a work of this kind than
are ever actually acknowledged. This is certainly the case
here. Over the past ten years I have had the great privilege
to work with two outstanding groups of staff, first at the
Maudsley Day Hospital and more recently in the
Cambridge Psychiatric Rehabilitation Service at Fulbourn
Hospital. Many of them have contributed to the development of my ideas, often possibly while being unaware
that they were doing so. I would like to express my grat-
itude and respect to them all. In addition, while a lecturer
at the Institute of Psychiatry I continually came into
contact with lively, intelligent students and colleagues who
helped sharpen my thinking and supplied me with many
new ideas. Finally, I have learned from many patients
what living with chronic psychological disabilities is really
like and their experiences have perhaps been the most
telling of all.

A few people deserve special mention. Rob Durham,
Steve Morley, Richard Mollica, Isobel Morris and Fraser
Watts are all friends and colleagues to whom I owe a great
deal. Simon and Sue, Laura and Jane also sustained me
during the writing of this book in their own very different,
but equally important, ways. I am grateful to the hospital
administration and my colleagues in the Psychology

Department for allowing me a short period of study leave during which the major part of the writing was completed. Rosemary Leech typed the manuscript beautifully. My series editor, Phil Feldman, patiently corrected the punctuation and healed the split infinitives and also made several helpful, additional suggestions. But, the contribution of one man is paramount. Douglas Bennett has been my inspiration and example, as he has been to so many people all over the world who are interested in the care of those with long-term psychological disabilities. I am sure that most of what is interesting and valuable in this book I learnt from him. The mistakes are all mine. It is with the greatest respect and affection that I would like to dedicate the book to him. He is the founder member – and indeed sole celebrant – of that exclusive circle of those who really *understand* what rehabilitation is about.

Geoff Shepherd
*Cambridge*

We are indebted to John Wiley & Sons Ltd for permission to use a case example by the author based on an article published in *Theory and Practice of Psychiatric Rehabilitation* edited by Fraser N. Watts & Douglas H. Bennett, pub. John Wiley & Sons, Chichester 1983.

# Chapter 1

# An introduction to psychiatric disability

This book is concerned with the care and rehabilitation of people with long-term psychiatric disabilities. We will consider their care in hospital from an historical perspective and also their care in the community which has been the more recent approach. In later chapters we will review some of the research which has addressed itself to the problem of understanding the relationship between organizational practices in long-term care settings and the interactions that take place there between staff and clients. We will then examine the whole process of organizational change in health services and finish with a discussion of some of the important issues for the future. Throughout the book we will draw upon the ideas and research findings of scientists and clinicians who have tried to understand these problems and to shed some light upon their solution. These are difficult and complicated problems with long histories and no one can claim to have solved them very adequately; however some fundamental principles have emerged. We have an idea of what doesn't work and why, we can recognize increasingly specific subgroups of the disabled and think about specific solutions suited to their needs, we have some kind of theory of what is important in long-term care and some guidelines for organizing services which follow from this. All these principles should become clearer as we go along.

Let us begin with some questions. Who are the psychiatrically disabled? How do they differ from people with other sorts of psychiatric and psychological problems? What is the size of the problem and the nature and course of psychiatric disabilities? What does 'rehabilitation' consist of? These are the issues to be addressed first. Before we start, a few words about terminology. The terms 'psychiatric illness', 'psychological disorder' and 'mental health' will be used more or less interchangeably. This is not meant to imply any underlying assumptions about medical diagnosis, aetiology, or the most appropriate methods of treatment. The term 'institution' will be used to refer to any formal organization or facility created to provide care for the psychiatrically disabled, whether or not it is actually a hospital in the narrow sense of the word. 'Rehabilitation' will be used to refer to the overall process of assessment, treatment and management of long-term disabilities and 'care' will be used in a more general sense to cover the totality of that which is offered by the helping services. The consumers of these services will be called patients, clients or people. Where the masculine pronoun is used it is for the sake of convenience only. No offence is intended.

## Who are the psychiatrically disabled?

Most of us are familiar with psychiatric or psychological distress in one form or another. Life is full of changes and disappointments, relationships go wrong, jobs are lost, people die and the results are often manifested in signs and symptoms of psychological disorders, albeit of a minor and transient kind. These are what Freud called in another context, 'the normal miseries of life'. But they are quite different from psychiatric disability. In this country, the bulk of psychiatric problems are presented to general practitioners, the commonest forms of these disorders being emotional disturbances (anxiety and depression). The patient is likely to receive some brief counselling – if they tell their doctor what is actually bothering them – and then a prescription for some kind of psychotropic medication (usually a minor tranquillizer or antidepressant). In 1977 there were nearly 30 million prescriptions dispensed by general practitioners for psychotropic drugs at a cost of over 30 million pounds (MIND 1980). Apart from the colossal cost involved this might be seen as a defensible strategy, since it is clear that approximately two-thirds of these patients will remit within six months even if they receive very little in the way of active treatment (Goldberg and Blackwell 1970). But, the psychiatrically disabled do not fall into this category. Their problems are more severe and more long-lasting. Indeed, they tend to get worse without active intervention rather than better. They are a very different group from the majority of psychiatric morbidity and they have very different characteristics and outcome.

This picture is illustrated if we follow a patient through the series of 'filters' between primary health care in the community (general practitioners, etc.), through psychiatric out-patient clinics, finally culminating in his/her admission to a mental hospital. This process is well described by Goldberg and Huxley (1980). It shows how, although there are different patterns of social correlates at each level (for example, a preponderance of women at the primary health-care level and a preponderance of men at the out-patient level) the most important single factor determining a patient's passage through the system is severity of his/her original disturbance (op. cit.: 133). Thus, at each level in the system it is only the most difficult cases who move on. By the time we come to the hospital we have therefore already focused on a highly selected group with particularly difficult problems. In social terms this group tends to contain larger numbers of single people and those from Social Class V (Cooper 1966). There are a number of reasons for this, but one factor is that people are more likely to come into hospital if they have no one else to look after them and limited means to support themselves outside. Once in hospital, a further filtering process takes place and the majority of cases are again successfully treated within a matter of a few months. After this, the chances of leaving hospital begin to decrease dramatically and after one year the prospects of discharge are very slim indeed. In 1976 less than 5 per cent of all discharges from mental hospitals in England and Wales had been in hospital for more than one year (MIND 1980). Therefore, those that remain join the residue of old 'long-stay' patients who form the bulk of our mental hospital population. In 1976 of the 83,939 in-patients in English psychiatric hospitals 68 per cent had been in hospital for more than one year and 46 per cent for more than five years. Nearly half of these were aged 65 or more. Those who have stayed in hospital for a very long time are now increasingly elderly and frail (Wing and Morris 1981).

We thus have a picture of psychiatric services as resembling a series of interconnecting rivers; each river corresponding to a different level or filter in Goldberg and Huxley's scheme. At each level there is a bulk of fast flowing water in the top of the stream with a murky sediment which settles to the bottom and gets passed down to the next level. This sediment gets progressively heavier as we pass down through the system, until we find ourselves eventually in the long-stay wards of the mental hospital. Here the most difficult and intractable problems reside. All the 'easy' cases have literally been filtered out and we are left with only the 'hard' ones. They are a daunting prospect indeed, so how can we begin to tackle them?

## What is psychiatric disability?

First, we must analyse the problem. After Wing (1978a) and Wing and Morris (1981) we can distinguish between three types of disability:
1. *Primary* (intrinsic) impairments, these usually consist of psychiatric symptoms.

2. *Secondary* handicaps, based on adverse personal reactions as a consequence of having been psychiatrically ill.
3. *Tertiary* (extrinsic) handicaps, consisting of social disablements which are either a consequence of the disturbance, or reflect pre-existing factors of deprivation and disadvantage.

The primary clinical impairments are the active pattern of symptoms which lead to diagnosis and the initial attempts at treatment. They are what takes the patient originally to hospital, although they are seldom the reason why he stays there. In diagnostic terms the bulk of those with long-term psychiatric disabilities are either suffering from schizophrenia or from some kind of affective disorder (depression, manic-depressive psychosis). These account, in roughly equal proportions, for about two-thirds of the total depending on the population surveyed. The remainder are a mixture of 'personality disorders', organic conditions (including drug abuse, alcohol), and dementias. Many of the patients have multiple disabilities, often with physical complications, e.g. high blood pressure, diabetes, etc. The primary symptoms may be disturbances of thinking, concentration or motivation (as in schizophrenia) or disturbances of emotional response (as in depression, or schizophrenia). In both cases various kinds of social and interpersonal difficulties may be present (withdrawal, hostility) and in both cases there is often a striking sensitivity to being upset by various life-events (Brown and Birley 1968). The secondary handicaps refer to the personal reactions which stem from the fact of having been ill, rather than the illness itself. A major psychiatric episode is a frightening and disturbing experience and its effects may persist long after the primary symptoms have disappeared. Characteristically, these reactions take two forms. Either the person loses confidence entirely and becomes wary of exposure to any kind of stress or challenge in case a further episode is precipitated. This avoidance can lead to a further loss of confidence and self-esteem until the person is so afraid to risk failure that he/she may be unwilling to do almost anything. In its extreme form, in hospital, this can lead to the apathy and withdrawal described as 'institutionalism' (Wing and Brown 1970) or the 'social breakdown' syndrome (Gruenberg 1967). On the other hand, the person may cope by denial, refusing to accept that they have any significant difficulties and clinging to fixed and unrealistic goals. In either case, these adverse personal reactions often present as much of a problem to rehabilitation as any primary symptoms. Finally, we have the tertiary, or extrinsic, handicaps. These are social disabilities such as poor family relationships, few friends, unemployment, poverty, etc. They can be seen either leading to the primary and secondary handicaps, or as a result of them. As we shall see later, there is some good evidence to suggest a strong continuity over time for these social handicaps and thus some reason to suppose that they may be seen as partly 'causal' of subsequent psychological disturbance (see Shepherd 1980; Shepherd 1983b). They are also more clearly the result of having been a psychiatric patient. Hence, the disruption to social relationships, the barriers to employment, 'stigmatization', etc., which all follow inevitably from having spent any length of time in a mental hospital and together constitute considerable problems for future adaptation.

This categorization of handicaps gives us a convenient way of analysing the difficulties of the long-term patient, but we must now look at these difficulties in more detail. Before that, we should consider the different groups of long-term patients and where they are to be found. So far we have focused on the long-term patient in hospital and sketched out the theoretical progression through which a new long-term patient is created. Of course, this theoretical progression is seldom followed in practice. In practice most patients, particularly the long-term ones find their way into hospital more or less directly through the hospital services themselves. Thus, they are already being followed up through out-patient clinics in the community, they then relapse and are readmitted. Two thirds of all admissions are thus readmissions (MIND 1980). The major 'gate-keeper' to the hospital is therefore the hospital itself. Only when the patient has been readmitted over and over again during a fairly short period of time, or when they remain on the admission wards for significantly longer than is usual, do questions begin to be raised about the possibility of long-term disabilities. There are therefore three possible groups of long-term patients:

1. *The old long-stay* – those who have been in hospital for a long time, and grown old there. As indicated earlier, many of these are also physically frail.

2. *The new long-stay* – new patients who are currently being added to the old long-stay population from the admission wards and from community follow-up. These are the new 'old long-stay' patients of the future and the rate at which they accumulate is a matter of considerable importance. Attempts to reduce this by providing services in the community, and an indication of the specialized provisions needed for them, will be described in Chapter 3.

3. *The new 'long-term'* – these patients cannot be called 'long-stay' as they are not necessarily staying in hospital. Instead, they are moving between hospital admission wards, day services, hostels, family homes, etc. Wing and Morris (1981) have suggested the name 'long-term' patients for this group, to reflect the extended and repeated nature of their contact. They estimate from the Camberwell Register that there were approximately 420 per 100,000 of the population in 1976 who had been in touch with the psychiatric services for more than a year. This would give a national estimate of around 210,000 people.

These three different groups have similar, but distinct, patterns of disability. In all cases the primary and secondary handicaps are prominent. However in the second, and especially the third, group (the new 'long-term') the social disablements as a consequence of illness may be less. The social disablements which are pre-existing are much the same. Thus, the new long-term patient is much like the old in terms of his symptoms, his personal difficulties in coping with illness and his premorbid history. However, he is different in the sense that he may have less of the social disablements that result from having been in hospital. The fact that he is main-tained for more of the time in the community, coupled with his sensitivity to life events, may also mean that he is rather more prone to symptomatic relapse. Let us now look at these disabilities in more detail.

## The nature of psychiatric disability

Different surveys of the old long-stay patients have tended to produce very similar results. For example, Christie-Brown et al. (1977) examined 220 patients in a large London mental hospital. The average age was 54 and approximately half the group fell into the 51–65-year-old age range. About three-quarters of the sample were men (this is a slightly higher proportion than usual and is partly attributable to local administrative factors). The group had an average length of stay in hospital of around 21 years and over a quarter had been in hospital for more than 30 years. Only a fifth of the sample had ever been married and only 7.7 per cent were still married. There was a preponderance of schizophrenics (67%). During the previous six months 55 per cent of the patients had not been visited and 80 per cent had not visited anyone outside the hospital, despite the fact that most of them were free to do so. In terms of other social disabilities, most of the patients were considered to require some sort of super-vised accommodation, although in only about a third of the cases was it felt that this actually needed to be in hospital. (The other alternatives were some kind of shel-tered setting similar to Part III accommodation for the elderly, or a long-stay hostel.) Only a very small number were considered to be able to cope with relatively independent living such as in a group home, with a landlady, or council housing. In terms of daily occupation, about a half of the patients under retirement age were considered to be capable of some kind of activity outside hospital although in this group, and more markedly in the over–65s, the presence of significant physical disabilities (nearly 20% overall) tended to restrict the range of daytime activities that were possible. This study has some methodological problems in that the judgements concerning accommodation and occupational needs were global ratings, made somewhat speculatively, and not based on direct observations. Nevertheless, they still provide a guide as to the needs of the old long-stay population. It is evident that we are faced with an elderly population, isolated from the outside world, who have grown old in hospital. Many of them may not need to be in hospital on clinical grounds, but in social terms there is a lack of suitable alternative places for them to go. They are now becoming increasingly elderly and physically frail. There is a need for more supervised accommodation, perhaps like Part III for the elderly, but for the majority of these patients it seems inevitable, and only right, that they should be allowed to remain in the hospital which has become their home until they die. The important question is, can we prevent the accumulation of another old long-stay population in another thirty years time?

The new long-stay have been investigated by Mann and Cree (1976). They began by selecting one hospital at random from each Regional Hospital Board in England and Wales. In each hospital patients who had been admitted for more than one but less than three years, and who were aged between 15–64 years, were then studied in detail. This involved 400 patients in all. In this sample the proportions of men and women were approximately equal, although there were most women in the older age group (55–64). Just over a half of the sample had been married, but only 19 per cent were still in contact with their spouse. In approximately 10 per cent of cases the marriage had apparently terminated during the current admission. About a quarter of the sample were living with parents prior to admission and a further 10 per cent with other relatives. There was evidence of marked occupational decline both between the patients' highest level occupation and their father's occupation, and between the patient's own peak level and the last employment before the current admission. Schizophrenia accounted for 44 per cent of the diagnoses and affective disorders about 16 per cent.

In terms of their social needs, about a third of the sample were considered to require further care in a hospital-type setting. This was mainly because of the presence of primary clinical symptomatology (usually schizophrenia). Another quarter were thought to need supervised accommodation, although not necessarily in hospital. This group tended to be poor at looking after themselves and in coping with the everyday tasks of living (shopping, washing clothes, paying bills, etc.). They appeared to require a considerable degree of supervision and prompting to prevent them lapsing into apathy and withdrawal. A further 15 per cent were thought to need much less supervised accommodation and the remainder (25%) were simply in hospital because there was nowwhere else for them to go. These patients tended to be suffering from organic conditions, or physical problems (16% overall). There was also an additional category of what the research team called 'asylum seekers'. These accounted for 5 per cent of the total and comprised individuals who had no clinical reason for remaining in hospital but simply preferred it to living outside.

Overall, just under a third of this sample expressed a strong desire to leave hospital and about the same proportions either expressed a strong desire to stay, or were apparently ambivalent. Previous studies (Wing and Brown, 1970) have shown that the desire to leave hospital tends to decrease with increasing lengths of admission, however Mann and Cree's study suggests that some long-term patients are ready to accept the hospital as their home fairly early on in their 'careers'. For them, 'institutionalization' is a product of acceptance rather than a result of coercion or control (a similar point has been made by Townsend 1976). Thus, they opt for life in hospital because they see it as most effectively meeting their needs and not because it is thrust upon them.

In terms of occupation, about a quarter of the sample appeared to be totally unoccupied. A further half did some kind of occupational or industrial therapy in the hospital, although often not on a regular basis. The remainder performed occasional work on the wards or helped around the hospital. Only 27 (7%) were employed outside. The research team considered that just over a quarter of the sample might be occupied in day care outside the hospital (13% in day centres; 7% in day hospitals and 6% in sheltered workshops).

This study also has some limitations. The judgements made as to need were reliable, but still essentially speculative. However, the conclusions are very similar to Christie-Brown et al. (1977). The new long-stay patient may have a range of possible psychiatric and physical impairments but only in a minority of cases are these sufficient to justify remaining in hospital. The majority are again likely to be in hospital for social, rather than clinical, reasons. They need someone to look after them, to supervise their needs, and to give them the necessary prompting to prevent them lapsing into apathy and inactivity. They have often become estranged from their families and have few social supports. Many prefer living in hospital because they perceive – probably realistically – that it may be better than most of the options outside. A number might benefit from day care outside the hospital if more of this were available.

The new long-term patients have not yet been as extensively studied as the other two groups, however we do know that they share many of the same handicaps. Thus,

Hewett et al. (1975) and Ryan and Hewett (1976) looked at new long-term patients living in a number of voluntary or local authority hostels in London. They noted the range of difficulties that these patients had in looking after themselves and, although they were often a highly selected group, they still required a very considerable degree of supervision simply to ensure that their daily needs were not neglected. One of the most striking disabilities of the group was the degree of social isolation that they manifested. A similar finding was reported by Wing and Creer (1980) who studied schizophrenic patients living at home with their families. They found that the most frequent characteristic, reported by 74 per cent of the families, was social withdrawal. Brown et al. (1966) also studied schizophrenic patients discharged from three mental hospitals over a five-year period and found that only two-thirds of the first admitted men, and one third of the previously admitted men, gained employment in this time. Over half of those unemployed at follow-up had done no work at all in the intervening period. (N.B. It should be noted that this study was conducted at a time when general unemployment levels were low.) More recently Ebringer and Christie-Brown (1980) examined two samples of newly admitted psychiatric patients and found that 65 per cent were unemployed at the time of admission. Of these, 77 per cent had been unemployed for more than a year. The majority of the patients were single and a quarter were currently living with their spouses; half were living alone at the time of admission. The picture of the new long-term patients is therefore very similar, to that of the new long-stay: they have problems in living, problems in work and problems in social relationships. These patients may have less of the 'tertiary' handicaps, i.e. they do not have the added burden of having spent twenty years in a mental hospital, but the primary and secondary handicaps are much the same, and the pre-existing social disabilities are also evident. So, what is the likely course and outcome of their disabilities?

## The course and outcome of psychiatric disabilities

The first and most obvious thing to say about long-term disabilities is that they do persist, i.e. they are 'chronic'. A chronic disability is one that has failed to respond given adequate treatment. (What constitutes 'adequate treatment' in a given case may be difficult to specify, but that is a problem we shall return to later, see pp. 19–20). Many of the psychiatric and social disabilities that we have been concerned with here may therefore show very little change over time. For example, we have noted repeatedly the low rates of marriage among long-term patients. This means that many of these patients may never have left their original parental homes, or lived independently, before their psychiatric problems began. Others may have come from disrupted home backgrounds and may already have spent periods in other institutions before coming into a mental hospital. In either case, they often lack many of the basic everyday skills necessary to look after themselves. These deficits were confirmed by observations such as Hewett et al. on the performance of long-term patients in hostels in the community. Regarding the longitudinal continuity of social disabilities, Neale and Ottmanns (1980) have also reviewed a considerable amount of evidence which suggests that children who go on to develop schizophrenic symptoms in later life show various kinds of social difficulties when young. Preschizophrenic boys are more likely to be aggressive and antisocial, whereas preschizophrenic girls tend to be more introverted and passive. (It should be emphasized that at the moment it is not clear whether such findings are specific to schizophrenia, or if they are more general prognostic signs of likely subsequent psychological disorder.) Prospective studies of social functioning such as Strauss and Carpenter (1974) confirm the strong relationship between social isolation, measured in the period before admission, and frequency of social contacts measured at two year follow-up. This research also showed the same relationship for regularity of employment in the year before admission and percentage of time employed in the follow-up period. Similarly, Watts and Bennett (1977) found that occupational stability in the first ten years of working life predicted successful return to work very well in a group of patients receiving vocational rehabilitation in the community.

All these studies point to one simple, and perhaps rather uncomfortable, fact: the past is often a very good guide to the future. This means that history *is* important, and that we cannot expect patients who have never functioned independently, or never sustained personal relationships, or never been able to hold down a job for any length of time, suddenly to be able to do so. Many show evidence of difficulties long before their psychiatric problems are actually manifest and they are likely to continue to show difficulties long after their actual 'symptoms' disappear. This is not to say that nothing ever changes, or that treatment is a waste of time, but we must provide services which are geared to accept the enduring nature of patients' disabilities and which set realistic goals. Examination of the course and outcome of disabilities also has some other implications.

Thus, in general terms it is well established that the lower the level of functioning prior to an illness episode the poorer the subsequent outcome is likely to be. This is especially true in schizophrenia (Zigler and Phillips 1961). However, Strauss and Carpenter's (1974) work mentioned earlier highlights the relative independence of different aspects of the outcome process. As indicated, premorbid social functioning tended to predict subsequent social functioning, premorbid employment record tended to predict subsequent employment, and duration of previous hospital admissions tended to predict future length of time in hospital. Outcome cannot therefore be thought of as a single process, rather it is a number of semi-independent outcome 'systems'. Strauss and Carpenter refer to this concept as the 'open-linked system'. (N.B. Since there is some degree of intercorrelation between the systems, there can be said to be some linking.) The implication is that different disabilities may change at different rates over time. Thus, Fontana and Dowds (1975) found that symptomatology, social integration and employment all had subtly different patterns of change over a six month period following admission. Fenton et al. (1982) reported similar results comparing groups of patients treated in hospital or mainly at home. As one might expect, symptoms tended to show the most rapid and steady improvements (they are the easiest to 'treat' directly) and social employment difficulties tended to improve more slowly, if at all, often leaving considerable residual disabilities even when the symptoms had almost completely recovered. These findings confirm our previous discussion of the patterns of disabilities observed in long-stay patients. The relative integrity of outcome systems over time also implies the necessity to provide services which are aimed at tackling each specific area of disability, and it further underlines the inadequacy of strictly medical, or symptomatic, models of care. Having looked at the nature, course and outcome of disability we are now finally in a position to examine the process of rehabilitation itself.

## What is psychiatric rehabilitation?

Douglas Bennett (1978a: 211) has defined rehabilitation as, 'the process of helping a physically or psychiatrically disabled person to make the best use of his residual disabilities in order to function at an optimum level in as normal a social context as possible'. He goes on to suggest that the success of rehabilitation should be judged by the extent to which the disabled individual is able to work independently, to sustain ordinary domestic and family responsibilities, and to make enjoyable and creative use of his leisure time. Rehabilitation is therefore concerned with maximizing functioning in various social roles. We have already described the kinds of problems that long-term patients have in coping with these roles and the further difficulties that long periods in a mental hospital may add. The long-term patient has few opportunities for normal role functioning and may effectively be presented with only one role: that of the chronic sick. This is a peculiar role and different from most others. If it is the only role available, then patients will soon lose the ability and desire to function in any other way. This is what chronic patienthood is, the loss of normal social roles and the substitution of the sick role. How does this process come about?

First, we must understand the nature of roles. The concept of role is relational, i.e. role performance can only be defined in relation to some person or reference group. Roles embody a set of consensual expectations about performance and behaviour and in this sense they can be said to be 'normative' (Secord and Backman 1964). It is therefore possible to specify, in broad terms, what is expected in particular roles. For example, someone living independently in the community is expected to be able to shop, cook, manage money, look after their clothes and themselves, occupy their leisure time, etc. Similarly, a 'worker' is expected to arrive more or less punctually, be occupied most of the time, accept supervision, chat with other workmates, ask for help, show initiative, take a joke, etc. A spouse is expected to show some evidence of love or affection for his or her partner, to contribute to the running of the home, and so on. But, as we attempt to unravel each set of role expectations, we soon run into difficulties. The skills necessary for successful role performance (instrumental, practical, social, emotional) can only be specified in very general terms and how these skills should be used in a specific context depends on the demands of the specific situation, i.e. the specific reference person or group involved. Thus, no two employers, or spouses, or friends have exactly the same role expectations. Therefore, in addition to the possession of certain practical skills we also need certain cognitive skills, for example a kind of empathy, an ability to judge which skills are appropriate in any given situation and when to use them. Successful role performance is therefore a very complicated process and this applies to all normal social roles with the possible exception of the 'sick role'.

The classic analysis of the sick role was performed by the sociologist Talcott Parsons (see Miles 1981: 54–60). He pointed out that its central characteristic is an exemption from some or all normal social responsibilities. For example, you are not expected to look after yourself if you are sick, you may be excused from domestic chores, you may not have to go to work, you may not even be expected to socialize. Furthermore, the sick person is not blamed for these deficits. They are ill and therefore they can't help it. These exemptions from performance and responsibilities apply equally, perhaps especially, to the mentally ill. However, as we have seen, psychiatric patients often stay in hospital long after their 'illness' has ceased to be a major problem; thus they are caught in a situation where the expectations are of 'sick role' behaviour, although the sickness is no longer present. Hence, they may be looked after when they can look after themselves, they may be excused from working when they are capable of work, their odd or socially unusual behaviour may be accepted and tolerated when it could be managed and reduced. All these expectations go together with being 'in hospital'; they are a part of the 'package deal'. Of course, the confusing thing is that they are sometimes justified. Sometimes the patient genuinely cannot meet normal social obligations and responsibilities, but these times are generally few and short-lived. The problem is how to make the system sufficiently sensitive such that it can respond quickly to changes in the patient's condition and thus ensure that sick role expectations are not perpetuated long after they are actually necessary. This is extremely difficult and, as we shall see in Chapter 4, this problem is not confined to the mental hospital. It can happen just as well in the 'community' if the same kinds of conditions are present.

Under such conditions it is not surprising that patients lose their abilities to cope with everyday social roles. But it is not just their abilities which suffer. In addition to abilities, successful role performance also depends on motivation. One must not only know what to do, and how and when to do it, one must also *want* to (Bennett 1978a: 213). Again, we saw earlier how various secondary handicaps (adverse personal reactions) can affect motivation, and hence performance. Thus, as well as losing skills the chronic patient may also lose motivation and, as Mann and Cree (1976) noted , this process can begin very early on in the patient's career. In this respect the chronic patient isn't even a 'good' patient for the only important motivational demand that the sick role makes is that the patient be motivated to get better. They should want to seek out treatment, to be co-operative and to leave hospital as quickly as possible. In many long-term psychiatric patients this is evidently not the case. They therefore run the risk of being labelled 'unmotivated', 'dependent', 'hysterical', 'manipulative', etc. Labelled in this way they may not even be deemed to be worth treating as 'patients', so what can be done with them then? Since they are 'untreatable', presumably they should be cared for by non-medical agencies, e.g. social services, voluntary organizations, prisons? This need to distinguish between those who are sick and therefore require treatment; and those who are simply deviant and therefore do not, is a deep theme in our culture. It has plagued care-givers and legislators ever since we changed our aetiological views about mental illness and began to suppose that it is, to some extent, under the individual's own control (rather than being caused by some external malevolence, or simply being a part of natural order of things). We shall return to this theme in the next chapter.

To return to rehabilitation, we are suggesting that it is simply concerned with helping those who have long-term psychiatric disabilities to cope with the tasks of everyday life as well as they can. To achieve this means providing them with the opportunities and the encouragement to perform social roles, in as normal a context as possible, and trying to maintain these roles. It will be immediately apparent that this is not easy in a mental hospital. For a number of sociological and historical reasons, hospitals often do not contain either the appropriate facilities, or the appropriate expectations. Since the patients' disabilities depend upon an interaction between their intrinsic difficulties and their environment, the extent to which the environment provides opportunities for normal role performance is crucial. It is therefore necessary to provide realistic settings where patients can look after themselves, work, and interact with others, in conditions which are as normal as possible. Their problems and difficulties can then be assessed by direct observation and treated where possible (see Shepherd 1983a). Since many of these problems may turn out to be untreatable, i.e. 'chronic', in the sense defined earlier, it will also be necessary to have a range of sheltered environments geared to different levels of disability which will maintain functioning, despite the presence of relatively fixed disabilities. This is what it is hoped to achieve through care in the community (see Ch. 3).

But, how can we tell when a disability is 'chronic'? How can we tell that adequate attempts at treatment have been made? Most therapists would probably argue that adequate treatment has not occurred until they themselves have had an opportunity to try. This is a laudable delusion, but it is also a recipe for frustration. In defining chronic disabilities a knowledge of the patient's history is obviously helpful (see pp. 13–15), but essentially the process has to be an empirical one. You can only try to treat the disability until you think you've tried hard enough and then look to maintaining functioning when it no longer seems possible to improve it. Treatment is therefore an integral part of the assessment process, helping to define the limits of chronicity. The important proviso is that one must always devote as much time and energy to maintaining functioning as to improving it. As we have seen there is an inherent tendency in the concept of the sick role to view untreatable patients as 'second-class' citizens.

Psychiatric rehabilitation is therefore very different from physical rehabilitation. In physical rehabilitation the emphasis is generally on treating symptoms, e.g. through drugs, physiotherapy, etc., and then making some relatively permanent adaptation by supplying some kind of physical prosthesis, e.g. an artificial limb or a wheelchair. This is possible because one is generally aiming at helping the disabled person to adapt to the physical world which is itself relatively stable. On the other hand, psychiatric rehabilitation has a much less strong treatment component (and treatments are much harder to carry out effectively) and a correspondingly stronger adaptation component, the adaptation being achieved through the provision of 'prosthetic environments', e.g. hostels, sheltered workshops, etc. Treatments are more difficult in psychiatry because one is not simply having to treat the person, one also needs to change the environment, particularly the social environment, if treatment effects are to persist. For the same reason the adaptation achieved will be more unstable. Adaptations to the social environment are bound to be more fragile since the social world is continually changing. People (staff, employers, friends, etc.) are continually coming and going and, as indicated at the beginning of this chapter, these life events have a profound effect on psychological adjustment, particularly for many long-term patients. It is as though a hemiplegic had to cope with a new wheelchair every six months! This temporariness of the outcome of psychiatric rehabilitation is often a difficult fact for staff to grasp. They tend to see it as a failure on their part (see Ch. 6). It is not. It is simply a reflection of the nature of psychological adaptation.

The adaptation achieved in psychiatric rehabilitation may be at a number of different levels, or at different levels in different areas. For example, in hospital or in the community; sheltered living and independent working, or independent living and sheltered working. This implies a range of services and individualized packages of care to suit each person's needs. There are many possibilities. Certainly, rehabilitation should not be seen as simply synonymous with discharge from hospital.

This view of rehabilitation as being concerned with adaptation may be contrasted with a 'ladder' model where patients are seen as being treated and then moving up successive rungs until they can be independent again. Since many of them never managed to live independently in the first place, the 'ladder model' has limited value. Emphasizing adaptation and de-emphasizing treatment also has other implications. For example, it means that treatment should not be seen as a 'one-off' exercise. Treatment techniques are important for defining the limits of disability and they may also contribute to long-term care and assist in the maintenance of functioning. Promoting long-term adaptation may therefore involve attempting to maintain a continuous state of treatment. This is a very different conception of long-term care from simple, passive custody. *Caring* is just as important and just as difficult as *curing*. It is unfortunate then that the latter is accepted as being the province of high status, highly qualified professionals, while the former can be left to those with neither status, nor qualifications (nor even, in many cases, adequate financial or emotional support).

To conclude, it is clear that psychiatric rehabilitation does not fit easily within a traditional medical framework. In particular, aspects of the 'sick role' and 'the treatment model' hold serious dangers for the long-term psychiatric patient. A more social model of care therefore seems appropriate. But, how can this be achieved? Before we try to answer this question, let us first examine how the present situation came about.

## Summary

People with long-term psychiatric disabilities constitute a very small proportion of the total psychiatric morbidity existing in a population at any one time. However, they are an important minority since their needs don't go away and they continue to make major demands on hospital beds and services. They suffer from a range of disabilities – psychiatric, physical and social – but the most important reasons for a continuing need for care tend to be social rather than clinical. Their difficulties can be best understood as a failure to be able to cope in various everyday social roles and rehabilitation can be seen as a process of helping them to do this as best they can. Rehabilitation is as much concerned with adaptation as it is with treatment and, for various reasons, it does not fit in easily within traditional medical concepts such as the 'sick role' and 'the treatment model'. A more social view of care is therefore recommended.

# Chapter 2

# Care in hospital

The philosopher George Santayana once said that those who cannot remember the past are condemned to repeat it. This remark is particularly apposite when we view the history of psychiatry. Ever since psychiatric patients emerged as a recognizable group a vast array of possible solutions to their problems have been tried. Many of these possible solutions have been tried more than once and many of the old themes have a remarkably contemporary ring about them. But history never quite repeats itself. Times and conditions change and solutions which were not acceptable, or even possible, 100 years ago may be possible today. One of the most interesting changes has been in our views as to the causes of mental illness and, we shall see later, as these have changed so have our ideas about what should be done for the mentally ill. But let us begin by describing the situation before the mental hospital existed.

## Before the asylum

Contrary to some popular belief the mental hospital is not a part of the natural landscape. Unlike the trees and the rivers it was put there by man, not by God. There was thus a time when mental hospitals did not exist; how did people manage then? Before the eighteenth century there was no clear definition of what mental disorder was and no clear recognition of the mentally ill as a separate category requiring a distinct form of care. Probably the first legislation one can point to which is relevant to the care of the mentally ill is the Elizabethan Poor Law Act of 1601. The main provisions of this act are described by Allderidge (1979) and essentially they consist of a mixture of what we might call today 'institutional' and 'community' care. Overseers of the poor were appointed in each parish and these usually consisted of prominent local figures, such as churchwardens or landowners. These people were charged with the responsibility to make provisions for the local poor and these provisions were basically of two types: 'outdoor relief' and workhouses.

The concept of 'outdoor relief' was an interesting one. It recognized that the pauper was unable to support himself and it therefore made provision to support him at home through parish funds, according to the means of the local community. (Hence his name might appear on the Poor Law Registers still seen today in many old churches.) The money might be paid direct to the pauper himself, or to his family or relatives if it was felt that he was unable, or could not be trusted, to manage his own affairs. We thus have an early example of a 'social service', maintained through local taxation, and based upon direct payments. An alternative model was to place the pauper with one of the local wealthy landowners and to provide accommodation and work on the estate. Allderidge quotes a number of examples of paupers being supported in this way and even being moved from house to house. The second type of Poor Law provision was the parish workhouse and again this was locally funded. Workhouses were there to provide work and, although conditions did vary from parish to parish, they were certainly generally rather harsh. The idea was to run the workhouses as cheaply as possible and to make them as unpleasant as possible so as to deter the able-bodied from using them. There was scant medical attention and no attempt was made to separate the mentally ill from other categories of the poor (with the possible exception of individual pioneering institutions like St Peter's workhouse in Bristol).

Thus, a situation had arisen where the mentally ill were simply lumped together with the rest of the poor: the old, the lame, the blind, orphans, single-parent families, anyone who could not look after themselves. They were then cared for, but only after a fashion. It is significant historically that the first attempts to provide for the mentally ill should have been through the Poor Laws. For the long-term mentally ill this close association with poverty therefore has a long history and, in many respects, it still holds true today.

Of course, for many pauper lunatics the provisions under the Poor Law constituted the least worst option. Thus, if they were not dealt with under the Poor Laws, they were likely to be dealt with under the criminal, or vagrancy, laws and their prospects were then possibly even more bleak. Our predecessors took a fairly pragmatic line concerning crime and there was no such concept as 'diminished responsibility' until well into the nineteenth century. The criminally insane were therefore sent to prisons or Bridewells (houses of correction). Conditions in these institutions are described briefly by Kathleen Jones (Jones 1972 21–4) and seemed fairly appalling. The inmates were regularly ill-treated, undernourished, often permanently chained, and deprived of basic amenities, even sometimes of fresh air, since their gaolers were often tempted to stop up the windows to avoid paying window tax. On top of all this, in prisons at least, the detained were required to pay for the privilege! They were responsible for their own maintenance and for the payment of gaoler's fees. (The latter did not generally receive a salary as did their counterparts in the Bridewells, which were partly administered by the Poor Law commissioners.) Brutality and degradation were thus the order of the day and if the offender continued to be a nuisance then more summary methods were available. There was certainly no idea of reform or rehabilitation and these concepts would have been meaningless to even the most enlightened minds of the seventeenth and early eighteenth centuries.

The Poor Laws were thus created in an attempt to respond to the flood of poverty which threatened to overwhelm Elizabethan England. The Vagrancy Laws were equally strict and contributed a high proportion of the admissions to gaols and Bridewells. The mentally ill figured large in the numbers caught up in both systems. But there gradually emerged a number of other alternatives. The first of these was the public (subscription) hospitals, the most famous of which the Bethlem, was founded in the thirteenth century (Guys, St Lukes and the St Bethel Hospital Norwich also have long histories). Conditions in the Bethlem have varied greatly over the centuries (Jones 1972). Perhaps some of the worst times are depicted in Hogarth's famous series engravings, *A Rake's Progress*, completed in 1733. Prior to that in the seventeenth century discharged patients were known as 'Tom O'Bedlams' and were given special badges which enabled them to beg so as to make up any arrears in fees that they owed. Unfortunately, as Jones notes, this often led to forging of the badges by less legitimate beggars wishing to gain the same privilege.

Although these public hospitals existed, their places were few and the contribution that they could make to the scale of the problem was very limited. A second alternative was therefore the private madhouse. These institutions grew quickly in number in the eighteenth and nineteenth centuries and their history is described in a classic book by William Parry-Jones entitled *The Trade in Lunacy* (1972). Private madhouses varied greatly in the conditions that they offered, some were undoubtedly caring and concerned, but others displayed a level of callousness and brutality which is almost incredible to us today. Most serious of all from the public's point of view was the fact that these institutions were not subject to any kind of outside scrutiny. This is the only safeguard against abuse that society has ever been able to devise and public concern over conditions in private madhouses, in particular the fear that sane people were being detained against their will, was the major factor leading to the reforms of the nineteenth century and the creation of the asylums. The private 'trade in lunacy' therefore stands as another important historical lesson, reminding us of the risks of exploitation of inarticulate and disadvantaged groups by organizations who are not publicly accountable.

The final provisions, and perhaps the most numerous of all, were the so-called 'single lunatics'. These were in the same tradition as the 'outdoor relief' of early Poor Law days. They comprised isolated individuals, cared for at home, and their numbers and the conditions under which they lived are not possible to estimate accurately. Certainly, they varied according to the family's attitudes and means from the mad uncle in the East wing, to the imbecile brother chained in a hut outside the village. The classic stereotype of the single lunatic is given by the Victorians, notably Charlotte Brontë in *Jane Eyre*. Here we have the picture of the unfortunate first Mrs Rochester, living in her deserted tower, presided over by a gin-soaked attendant. The picture is not exactly a sympathetic one and it reveals the public attitude towards the mentally ill of fear mixed with prurient interest, an attitude which is still common today. The single lunatics – like the poor – have therefore been with us a long time, and again we are reminded that although families may be willing to care for their afflicted members there are possible dangers involved.

From this brief review it is clear that for some hundreds of years the use of a medical model in the care of the mentally ill was minimal. The involvement of medical ideas such as 'illness' and 'treatment' are thus relatively recent innovations. There are a number of reasons for this. In the first place medicine was, until well into the nineteenth century, not an entirely reputable profession. Standards were low and knowledge rudimentary. Practice dominated largely by the Galenic ideas that illness was caused by an imbalance of one of the four basic bodily humours (blood, bile, phlegm and choler). Treatments consisted therefore mainly of attempts to restore the balance by bleeding, purging and emetics. These methods, combined with the widespread use of mechanical restraints (manacles, chains, strait-jackets, etc.) consti- tuted the main 'therapies' on offer to the mentally ill from the medical profession. Not surprisingly many patients and their relatives preferred to steer well clear of doctors believing – perhaps with some justification – that the cure might be worse than the disease. But doctors were also working within a cultural context in which the popular ideas concerning the aetiology of mental illness empha- sized demonic possession, witchcraft, the fall from Grace, or simply accepted the ill and disabled as an inevitable part of the natural order of things. It was therefore logi- cal that the care of the mentally ill should proceed on the basis of simple custody. If the causes were beyond their power to influence, what point was there in trying to treat the symptoms? This tendency to ignore the mentally ill was reinforced by the public's fear of insanity which was itself fuelled by their fear of mistaken incarceration. Mental illness was thus seen as a social and legal prob- lem, but not a medical one. The legal theme was to continue, but the social one became lost, at least temporarily.

The failure to distinguish the mentally ill as 'sick' has been seen by some as a failure in the Poor Law legislation. Because they were not defined as such they were deprived of the 'benefits' of treatment. As we have seen this was often not such a great disadvantage, but it had some other interesting implications. For example, it removed the necessity to decide between those who *could not* support themselves and those who *would not*. This meant that it prevented a division into those who were sick and there- fore deserved treatment; those who were disabled and therefore deserved care and those who were neither sick nor disabled, but simply lazy, and therefore deserved nothing. Care was thus defined according to need and not according to some dubious judgement of aetiological or moral 'cause'. This useful principle has been lost today. Why?

## Enlightenment, moral treatment, and the invention of the asylum

Towards the end of the eighteenth century and the beginning of the nineteenth there took place throughout Europe and America what has been called the 'Age of Enlightenment'. The divine rule of kings was challenged, governments toppled and everywhere established ideas and existing orders were threatened. Out of this ferment grew a generation of political and social reformers (Rousseau, Paine, Bentham, Mill) whose ideas and philosophies were to have a profound impact on the outlook of ordinary people. Most important in this change of public opinion was the idea that social problems might be caused by the societies that contained them. Social problems were no longer seen simply as the result of some external malevolence, or divine will, but as the product of defective social structures. If these social structures could be perfected then the problems should disappear. This strand of thinking passed down directly to the Victorian reformers and, of course, eventually to Marx and Engels and the revolutionaries of the twentieth century. For our purposes it is the effect that they had on attitudes to mental illness that is important. People began to suggest that mental illness might have environmental rather than internal causes and therefore that if the right kind of environment could be created, mental illness might be 'treatable' after all. David Rothman has argued that it was this shift in aetiological belief which contributed most significantly to the invention of the asylum (Rothman 1971). He also argues that a similar trend can be seen in the growth of penal institutions.

Of course, there were other factors. Jones (1972)

describes the impact in England of the prolonged illness of King George III. Whether this was due to advanced syphilis or porphyria is unclear, but it was certainly a *mental* illness of some sort. Thus, in the public mind, mental illness was something that could happen to anybody, even a king. In addition, the combined efforts of the King's doctors to treat his condition (complicated by the political overtones to the whole affair) strengthened the impression that mental illness might be, in principle, curable. There was also the growing concern, mentioned earlier, over conditions in the private madhouses. This led to an Act regulating their conduct in 1774 and a Select Committee report in 1816. Finally, there were changes in the Vagrancy Laws which slowly began to reflect a recognition that some vagrant and poor people might not be simply indolent and might require special forms of care and treatment. All these changes culminated in attempts to create humane and therapeutic conditions in institutions specifically set aside for the mentally ill. Lunatic asylums were therefore founded on the basis of therapeutic optimism. They were not originally brought into being as safe havens where the deviant and disorderly of society might be dumped and quietly forgotten. Instead, they were conceived of as advanced social environments where, through the provision of a refuge from the stresses and strains of an obviously corrupt society, the mentally ill might be reformed and rehabilitated to a more productive life. This period has been termed the 'Moral Treatment Era' (Bockoven 1963).

In England, one of the foremost pioneers of the new approach was William Tuke, founder of the York Retreat. This was begun in 1792 and the name 'Retreat' was chosen so as to designate it as neither a hospital nor an asylum. Tuke wished it to be, 'a quiet haven in which the shattered bark might find the means of reparation or of safety'. The York Retreat was a small institution, built to accommodate only thirty patients, and all its residents – or 'family' as Tuke preferred to call them – came from generally well-to-do backgrounds. It was not intended to provide for the pauper insane. The principles of 'moral management' were, as Kathleen Jones so aptly puts it, 'based not on the scanty medical knowledge of the time, but on Christianity and common-sense' (Jones 1972: 45). Tuke believed that patients could be rational and controllable provided they were not aggravated by cruelty, hostility or harsh methods of restraint. Mechanical restraint was kept to a minimum and patients were not punished for failure to control their behaviour, rather certain amenities were given to them in order to foster self-control by a show of trust. Every attempt was made to occupy the inmates, they were given animals to care for, they helped in the garden, the women knitted or sewed and writing materials and books were provided. Tuke was a devout Quaker and so there were also regular religious services. The York Retreat became a model for the new approach to mental illness and by 1808 the first County Asylums Act had been passed encouraging local communities to fund and build their own lunatic asylums.

The asylum movement was initially slow to gain momentum, probably at least partly because local people were reluctant to spend three times as much money in caring for patients in the asylum as it cost in the work-house. However, fuelled by another series of scandals concerning conditions in mental institutions, gradually the pressure began to build up for reform. The medical profession was also beginning to change its ideas. Dr Charles-worth, a physician at the new Lincoln asylum, introduced a policy of 'non-restraint', i.e. not using mechanical devices to hinder patients' movements. This was taken up by a Mr Robert Gardiner Hill the house surgeon who in 1838 claimed to have totally abolished the use of personal restraint. There then followed an acrimonious public debate between the two doctors as to who should have the credit for these advances. Dr John Conolly was also made physician superintendent at the newly created Hanwell asylum in 1839 and he, influenced by the events at

Lincoln, began to eliminate the forcible restraint of patients. He also introduced educational classes for the patients and began a training scheme for attendants and young doctors in the management and treatment of the mentally ill. An indication of the shift in public and medical attitudes is given by the Appendix to the Select Committee report 1827 (reproduced by Jones 1972: 106–7). Here we see a clear statement of expected standards of care and those interested might like to compare them with Appendix D to the Nodder Report (DHSS 1979). Paraphrasing the Commissioners' words, they required to know:

1. *On accommodation*. Are the dormitories properly ventilated? Are there complete baths?
2. *On physical care*. What steps are taken to ensure the personal cleanliness of the patients, particularly the most unclean? How often is bathing insisted upon? Is there daily exercise?
3. *On occupation*. How far has manual labour been adopted? Has the active engagement of the mind to the science, fine arts, literature or mechanical arts been attempted with patients of a superior description, and what has been the result? Where graver studies would be unsuitable, what of drawing, painting, designs, models, gardening, etc.? Where the mind is so diseased as to be evidently unfit for the foregoing exercises, has benefit been experienced by furnishing the patients with means of innocent amusement, music, domestic animals, poultry, birds, flowers and objects of a similar nature? Is it the opinion of the superintendent that a state of entire indolence and mental inertness is decidedly prejudicial to the patient?
4. *On moral treatment*. Is it considered an object of importance to encourage their own efforts of self-restraint in every possible way, by exciting and cherishing feelings of self-respect? And, by generally maintaining a treatment uniformly judicious and kind, sympathizing and at the same time diverting their

minds from painful and injurious associations?

At the same time, similar developments were taking place in America. Pliny Earle, a physician superintendent of the 1840s makes a clear statement of the principle of 'normalization', viz. 'The primary object is to treat the patients, so far as their conditions will possibly admit, as if they were still in the enjoyment of the healthy exercise of their mental faculties' (quoted in Bockoven 1963: 69). Bockoven goes on to describe the main principles of moral treatment; they included:

1. The acceptance of a continuum between sanity and insanity. The mentally ill were not to be seen as belonging to a qualitatively separate category.
2. The insane could be understood by gaining a thorough knowledge of their history and background and of their 'inner life' (hopes, fears, etc.).
3. This could only be achieved through sympathy and compassion, hence the importance of carefully selected and trained attendants.
4. Positive encouragements should be used rather than punishments.
5. The patient's care should be explained to him together with the reasons why things were being done.
6. In general, an attempt should be made to create a well-ordered and homely environment, like a good family. Staff should mix freely with the patients and on an equal footing, patients should be encouraged to help one another.
7. The asylum is important as a refuge, to protect the patient from the stresses and strains of modern life. It should therefore be situated well away from the industrial towns, which were corrupt and polluted.
8. It is important to avoid monotony and boredom. Patients should be given work and education to engage and distract the mind. (Dr Earle gave a series of lectures on astronomy, physiology, chemistry, aesthetics, poetry and the history of Greece and Malta before 1838!)

These principles have a strong flavour of Victorian paternalism, the sanctity of the family, the value of work, etc.; but, nevertheless, they embody a set of desirable minimum standards. It is something of a tragedy to see how quickly they were eroded. In 1845 the new Lunatics Act was passed making it compulsory for counties to provide Asylums and there followed both in England and America a great period of hospital building. Nearly all our mental hospitals were built at this time (indeed it sometimes seems that they all had the same architect). Standards were good and hopes were high, however barely thirty years later in 1877 a commission of doctors sponsored by the medical journal the *Lancet* was worried that conditions in the new asylums were already beginning to deteriorate. By the early part of the twentieth century after the First World War had taken its toll, another doctor, Montagu Lomax, again drew the public's attention to the drab and inhumanitarian conditions in mental hospitals (Lomax 1921). So, what went wrong? Why did conditions deteriorate so much, and so rapidly? History is always difficult stuff to be sure of, but we can identify some of the factors.

## The decline of hospital care

Kathleen Jones, on whom I have drawn extensively in this chapter, argues strongly that one of the major reasons for the decline in hospital care was the triumph of legalism over medicine. The public became increasingly worried, as indeed it always had been, by the spectre of being illegally detained in a mental institution. It must be appreciated that, in the nineteenth century, virtually all hospital treatment could only be given after certification. This may be contrasted with the situation today where over 90 per cent of patients have informal status. It must also be noted that although the public were frightened of wrongful detention in a mental institution, this did not necessarily mean that they objected to conditions there. They simply did not wish to experience them themselves. This fear of mistaken incarceration led to a preoccupation with legal safeguards culminating in the Lunacy Act of 1890 (Jones 1972: 176–81). She suggests that the restrictions of this Act had a profound effect on medical and social practice in the institutions for the next seventy years.

The 1890 Act made it effectively impossible for the asylums to deal with early diagnosis and treatment of the mentally ill. Thus, although ideas of 'community care' and 'prevention' were already being voiced in the late nineteenth century (for example, the work of the Mental After-Care Association founded in 1879) the main advances in the treatment of mental illness took place outside the mental hospital and were concerned with outpatient care and the treatment of neuroses (for example, the development of psychoanalysis and the out-patient facilities at the new Maudsley hospital, see p. 37). The rules of certification in the Act were so heavily weighed against making a 'false positive' decision that the patient had to be so obviously mad they were more or less beyond hope. This left hospitals with only the most difficult and chronic cases and undoubtedly contributed to the re-emergence of custodial attitudes. In addition to demoralizing staff, it also meant that institutions were less likely to attract bright, ambitious, young doctors interested in making a name themselves by advancing the care of the mentally ill. Psychiatry has always been a low status profession in comparison with the rest of medicine and this is possibly a part of the reason. Without good staff, standards are bound to suffer.

A second major reason for the decline of mental hospitals was size and overcrowding. In 1827 the average number of patients per asylum was 116, in 1870 it was 542, in 1900 it was 961 and by 1930 it had risen to a staggering 1,221. The proportions of persons receiving in-patient treatment reached a peak in 1914, at 3.77/1,000 of the population. (The current guideline of in-patient beds is 0.5/1,000.) This enormous increase in size, which was mostly created by the migration of poor people from the country to the towns as a part of the growing process of industrialization, led to overcrowding on a terrible scale. It followed that the principles of moral treatment, which were fundamentally based on a recognition of the patient's individuality and the creation of a homely atmosphere, were no longer possible to put into practice. Dr Granville of the *Lancet* commission of 1877 was already saying at the time of conditions in Hanwell, that 'the treatment is humane, but it necessarily lacks individuality, and that special character which arises from dealing with a limited number of cases directly . . . it is only in a small asylum that this potent remedy, the sane working quietly, patiently and directly, can be brought to bear on individual cases' (Jones 1972: 227).

A third reason, and the one which is particularly advocated by Bockoven (1963) and Rothman (1971), was yet another shift in the prevailing aetiological views. As it became evident that the early hopes for curing mental illness through institutional means were over-optimistic, so a disillusionment with 'treatment' began to set in. This disillusionment was reinforced by the apparent accumulation of chronic and 'incurable' cases. Staff felt that if treatment was impossible then the only option was simple custody. They found it difficult to accept a concept of active care, or the necessity of maintaining a continuous state of treatment so as to prevent deterioration (cf. pp. 20–1). This view was further reinforced by the discovery in 1890 of the spirochete basis to tertiary syphilis. Since syphilis had been virtually endemic throughout Europe and America and constituted a major threat to physical and mental health, the discovery of a physical cause had a profound effect. Scientific medicine was now establishing itself and many people believed it was only a matter of time before all the other psychological problems yielded their physical secrets. Some people still believe this. The effect a hundred years ago was to persuade many doctors, politicians and administrators that the only sensible thing to do was to provide a basic level of physical care for the mentally ill and wait for science to come up with the answers.

All these factors worked together and it is impossible to separate out their effects, however the outcome was that conditions in mental hospitals undoubtedly deteriorated. The positive aspects of moral treatment disappeared and all that was left were large numbers of patients being kept in strict order in huge, remote asylums. We now have to look into the twentieth century to see the emergence of the next set of ideas that were to hold sway.

## Into the community

As indicated above, the period around the turn of the century was when mental hospitals achieved their status as the 'backwaters' of the health service, but out in the main stream things were happening. Henry Maudsley (John Conolly's son-in-law) offered the London County Council £30,000 to build a new mental hospital. It was to deal exclusively with early and acute cases, to have an out-patient clinic and to provide for teaching and research into mental illness. In 1915 the hospital bearing his name was opened. The Maudsley was also the first hospital to treat non-certified patients, a move which had been recommended by the *Lancet* commission back in 1877. It reflected the growing interest in neurotic conditions and in the new forms of psychological treatment such as psychoanalysis. These exciting developments in the care of psychological problems were to do much to change public attitudes. Indeed, nowadays going to see one's psychotherapist has almost become a status symbol; in America, psychotherapy and psychoanalysis have come to almost dominate the mental health services. But, all this energy and activity did little to impinge on the patients or conditions in mental hospitals.

Similar developments were taking place with regard to

the concept of 'prevention'. The authors of the minority report of the Poor Law Commission of 1909 (Sidney and Beatrice Webb) had already stressed the importance of public health measures in preventing illness, whether physical or mental, and the Royal Commission on Lunacy and Mental Disorder of 1924–26 suggested that, 'the keynote of the future must be prevention and treatment'. To this end they saw the development of out-patient and after-care services as paramount. Their thoughts on this matter are strikingly similar to modern views, viz., 'The transition from asylum life to the everyday world is a stage of peculiar difficulty for the recovered patient. The home and family life to which he returns may be unsuitable or unsympathetic; employment may be hard to obtain, and friends may be unable or unwilling to help' (Jones 1972: 242). In 1929 the first English course to train social workers was founded at the London School of Economics and in 1930 the first school for occupational therapists at Dorset House in Bristol. Up until the outbreak of the Second World War the developments in out-patient and after-care continued, encouraged by the 1930 Mental Health Act, and although the war led to loss of staffing and overcrowding – as the first war had – in general these attempts to improve the mental health services proceeded. However, it was still the case that the major changes had taken place outside the mental hospital rather than within it.

After the war the situation was again different. There was a new generation of young, radical social psychiatrists and they shared an aversion to 'institutions' of all kinds. Memories of the war and concentration camps were still fresh in people's minds and the concept of institutional care came to have a distinctly pejorative ring about it. Goffman began his studies of the 'total institution' (see Ch. 4) and by that time the desire for more humane conditions in institutions was being reflected by the establishment of 'open-door' policies and therapeutic communities (see Jones 1968; Clark 1974). This desire was further strengthened in Britain by the establishment of a National Health Service in 1948.

The story of the National Health Service is vividly told by Michael Foot in his biography of Aneurin Bevan (Foot 1975). It was controversial from its inception and Bevan had a famous and protracted dispute with the medical establishment who saw it as threatening 'medical freedoms'. But it did survive, and the principle upon which it was founded ('bread for all before cake for anybody') had enormously important implications for the care of the mentally ill. Bevan wrote that, 'No society can legitimately call itself civilized if a sick person is denied medical aid because of lack of means' (Foot 1975: 1973). For the mentally ill this meant that the National Health Service attempted to heal the growing rift between poor people with major psychiatric illnesses who tended to be looked after in hospital, and wealthier people with less severe conditions who were looked after in the community. It was hoped that by providing a single administration for general practitioners, out-patients and hospital services this would prevent the growth of a 'two-tier' system for mental health. Consistent with this was an emphasis on after-care and prevention and a desire to encourage local authorities to provide for the mentally ill. It thus acted as a forerunner to the 1959 Mental Health Act (see below) and the reorganization of Social Services following the Seebohm report of 1968. While all these aims were by no means perfectly realized, much has been achieved. It is certainly the case that our mental health services show less of a sharp division between hospital and community care than do many other countries such as America (see Bennett 1973).

There was one other important factor which contributed to changes in mental hospitals and this was the introduction of major tranquillizers (chlorpromazine, phenothiazine, etc.). These were in widespread use by the mid-1950s, but writers like Wing (1978b) have noted how many of the progressive policies to liberalize conditions in mental hospitals had already begun before their introduction.

The interpretation of historical events is difficult, and once again we cannot say with any degree of certainty whether it was the social, administrative or pharmacological changes that were the most important. However, a new climate of opinion had been achieved and an influential report of the World Health Organization in 1953 reflected this in a new model for mental health services. The 'classical' system, they said, was one in which the mental hospital dominated the service, operating virtually a closed system and controlling any services in the surrounding community. The 'modern' system was to be one in which a variety of services – in patient, out-patient, day care, domiciliary care, hostels and so on – operated as 'tools' in the hands of the community, and the hospital became only one tool at the disposal of the medico-social team (see Jones 1972: 293). This new concept was to be developed slowly in the succeeding years, helped on its way by the 1959 Mental Health Act which encouraged even more treatment on a voluntary and informal basis, introduced various other safeguards over patients' rights and permitted local authorities to develop their own services for the mentally ill to complement those of the health authorities. Most of all the Bill embodied a principle of reorientation of services away from hospital care towards care in the community. How far we have actually progressed down this road will be examined in the next chapter.

However, before we leave the history of institutional care, a few words should be said in defence of the medical profession. In recent years doctors have become fashionable targets for the 'anti-psychiatry' movement. However, unfortunately this has often missed the point. Writers like Treacher and Baruch (1981) suggest that the history of psychiatry is a history of a profession intent upon securing medical hegemony over the psychiatrically disadvantaged, in order to use this position to repress and control the socially deviant. This seems neither fair, nor accurate. While it is true that doctors gradually emerged as the most powerful single profession in the mental health services, the extent to which one sees this as evidence of a sinister motive at work largely depends upon the extent to which one believes in a conspiracy theory of history. Would one make the same allegation concerning teachers and education? Is it simply an anti-professional stance? It is certainly not the case that doctors have been uninvolved in reforms within mental health services and we have documented numerous instances from the Charlesworth–Gardiner Hill controversy of the 1830s to the WHO report of 1953. Of course, doctors do tend to be 'establishment' figures. Is this their real 'crime'? As for suggesting that psychiatry has done little to promote, 'the goal of a society truly fit for human habitation' (Ingleby 1981: 45) I, for one, would be most worried if such an aim were to be seen as being the responsibility of the medical profession. I am jealous of my political rights and I would be reluctant to concede them to any one professional group.

Notwithstanding these objections, it is true that medical *concepts* have had a profound, and sometimes retrogressive, effect on the care of the mentally ill (as have legal ones). The dominance of the 'sick role' and the 'treatment model' (see Ch. 1) have contributed to poor quality institutional care. The pre-eminence of 'treatment' has also led to a diversion of attention and resources away from the chronically disabled and the 'untreatable'. But these ideas are often held just as vigorously by non-medical professionals. It is therefore medical *ideas*, not the medical *profession* which need to be challenged. It is then ironic that these critics of psychiatry should themselves espouse the most elite treatment of all, namely psychoanalysis (see Ingleby 1981: 61–71).

## Summary

The care of the long-term mentally ill has strong links with the care of the poor. Progress has been slow and uneven, nevertheless the mentally ill have gradually emerged as a recognizable group requiring distinct forms of care and treatment. Aetiological views have changed and as we have shifted more towards medical and treatment models so the importance (and difficulties) of providing good quality care have been undervalued. There has been a fall and rise of ideas concerning the importance of care in the community as opposed to care in institutions, although the mental hospital itself was founded with great therapeutic optimism. The decline in the quality of institutional care was associated with increasing size, overcrowding and disillusionment. There has also been a strong pressure from time to time for legal safeguards to protect individual liberties and these have sometimes worked against the advantage of patients. The current patterns of community care were made possible through changes in social attitudes, the establishment of a National Health Service and the introduction of major tranquillizers.

# Chapter 3

# Care in the community

In 1961, the then Minister of Health, Enoch Powell, delivered a famous speech to the Annual Conference of the National Association for Mental Health. In his own inimitable style he described this country's mental hospitals, 'isolated, majestic, imperious, brooded over by the gigantic water-tower and chimney combined rising unmistakable and daunting out of the countryside'. But he went on to make a startling revelation,

> I have intimated to the hospital authorities who will be producing the constituent elements of the national hospital plan that in fifteen years time there may well be needed not more than half as many places in hospitals for mental illness as there are today. Expressed in numerical terms, this would represent a redundancy of no fewer than 75,000 hospital beds (MIND, 1961).

Just for once the Minister meant exactly what he said. In 1954 there were approximately 150,000 patients resident in mental hospitals in England and Wales, in 1979 there were 76,000. The proposed reduction by half had been almost exactly achieved. Thus, whatever else one might say about 'community care' it is no longer a slogan. It is a reality. Whether the reality can be made to work to the benefit of the patients involved is another question and this is what will concern us in the next two chapters.

## What is 'community care'?

We saw in the previous chapter how people gradually became interested in shifting the balance of care for the long-term mentally ill back towards the community and away from the hospital. Care in the community thus consists of attempting to provide as many services as possible, for as many patients as possible, from a community rather than a hospital base. Hence, we should be careful to distinguish between 'care *in* the community' and 'care *by* the community'. The community must not be expected to provide care by itself. This would place an unrealistic responsibility on families, voluntary organizations, etc., and while it is necessary, indeed desirable , that informal care-givers should make a significant contribution to the care of the long-term mentally ill they should not be asked to accept intolerable burdens. The statutory authorities (health and social services) must provide the core of the services around which the informal agencies can make their supplementary contributions. But, what should these core services consist of? To answer this question we need to go back to the mental hospital and examine in detail the services that it provided.

Bachrach (1976, 1978) in an important series of articles has analysed the 'deinstitutionalization' movement of the 1970s in America. She makes the point that the original polarization of views for and against 'hospital' or 'community' has slowly disappeared and there has been a growing acceptance of the complementarity of hospital and community services. Nevertheless, there is still a strong desire to move away from the hospital base wherever this is possible. To achieve this, Bachrach (1978: 20–1) suggests that we must understand very clearly the manifest and latent functions that the hospital served. These include:

1. *A recognition of the necessity for long-term care.* As indicated in Chapter 1 an appreciation of the course and outcome of psychiatric disabilities is a necessary

prerequisite for providing an adequate service to meet their needs. If the mental hospital did nothing else, at least it provided long-term care.

2. *Asylum (a place of refuge) for both patients and their families*. The concept of asylum has occupied a central role in the history of the mental hospital (see pp. 29–34). Thus, providing a place of refuge for patients from the stresses and strains of living with their families and coping with life 'outside' is a crucial function. Similarly, providing families with relief from the stresses and strains of living with patients and coping with life 'outside' is an equally important function. As we shall see later, this need for asylum can usually be provided effectively without the need to resort to in-patient admission.

3. *Accommodation*. At its most basic level the mental hospital provided shelter, a bed and food (and did so cheaply).

4. *Medical treatment*. The mental hospital also provided medical treatment for both psychiatric and physical problems although, due to a shortage of doctors among other things, this was often not of a very intensive or adequate kind.

5. *Social and vocational help*. Again, depending on local circumstances some mental hospitals also provided a degree of help with social and vocational disabilities (through psychological treatments, occupational therapy, etc.). Once again, this was sometimes not a very satisfactory kind (Wing and Brown 1970).

6. *Custody*. Mental hospitals, ever since the days of the Bridewells, have provided an alternative placement for that group whom Gunn (1977) has referred to as a 'stage army', social misfits who shuffle miserably between prisons, hospitals and the gutter. Mental hospitals thus provided a degree of supervised accommodation for psychiatric patients who also have criminal problems.

7. *The illusion of a comprehensive service*. Bachrach

(1976: 20) notes that mental hospitals provided a place for, 'siphoning off the least affluent and least attractive of the mentally disturbed . . . creating the illusion that all local mental health needs are being met'. This 'illusion of comprehensiveness' is an important feature of the mental hospital system and we need to think carefully as to how it might be preserved.

8. *Secure employment for a range of mental health professionals*. Finally, the mental hospital provided employment. This is not to be overlooked as the most powerful forces resisting change in mental health systems will always come from the professionals working within them (see Ch. 5).

It is an impressive list. The question we must now ask is, can these functions be met in other ways? Care in the community begins with a considerable advantage since it does, by its very nature, break up what Goffman (1961) referred to as the 'total institution'. Goffman (1961: 17) noted that, 'A basic social arrangement in modern society is that the individual tends to sleep, play and work in different places, with different co-participants, under different authorities, and without an overall rational plan. The central feature of total institutions can be described as a breakdown of the barriers ordinarily separating these three spheres of life.' Community care locates sleep, play and work in different places and can therefore help to fragment the total institution. However, it still needs a community base to work from. This is where day care comes in.

## Day care

As Bennett (1981a) has suggested day services provide the cornerstone of community care. They can provide an alternative to in-patient admission and long-term care in hospital and an effective method of after-care, easing the transition from 'asylum life to the everyday world' (cf. p. 38). In this country, day care is provided mostly by health authorities (75%) and to a lesser extent by social services (20%). There is also a small contribution from the voluntary sector. (Figure quoted from the National Day Care Project in Edwards 1981; Edwards and Carter 1979.) The separation between health and social services provision has proved a difficult one. Originally, the health authority units (day *hospitals*) were conceived of as providing facilities for treatment and a range of occupational and rehabilitation activities, while the social services units (day *centres*) provided 'help in difficulties with forming or maintaining personal relationships, adjusting or readjusting to the demands of work and encouraging a realization of the individual's potential' (DHSS 1975). This somewhat confused statement seems to strive towards a distinction between a medicals/ treatment model (health services) and a social/care model (social services). In practice some separation of function has been achieved, although there is still a considerable degree of overlap. Thus, Edwards and Carter found that the day centres tended to deal with a rather more chronic population, containing more men, and more schizophrenics and seemed to be more concerned with longer-term maintenance; day hospitals tended to contain more women, more people reporting depressive symptoms, and seemed to be more concerned with acute treatment. To a large extent this difference may reflect the different staffing patterns in the two kinds of units (Edwards and Carter 1979: 44) there being on average more than twice as many staff in the day hospitals compared with day centres (staff/patient ratios in day hospitals are 1:3.5; in day centres 1:8.) and many more qualified staff, particularly nurses. A higher concentration of 'treatment-oriented' staff inevitably leads to a greater emphasis on this component, almost irrespective of the characteristics of the patients. (It is revealing in this comparison that units set up to provide 'care' should only be deemed worthy of a half of the staffing of units set up to provide 'treatment'.)

This brings us on to the question of for whom day services should be providing and how they fit into the overall pattern of care for the long-term mentally ill. As indicated above, they can either be seen as an alternative to admission for acute cases, or as a transitional facility to ease the move back into the community following a period of in-patient care; we can now add a third function, that of providing long term support and maintenance. Each of these functions is relevant to the care of the long-term mentally ill. Thus, as described in Chapter 1, although the majority of acute psychiatric admissions get better and leave hospital fairly quickly, there will still be a proportion who prove difficult to discharge or who, once discharged, keep returning. This group of 'chronic-acute' cases represent some of the new long-term cases in the community and informal surveys suggest that they may constitute up to a third of those currently resident on admission wards at any one time (Shepherd 1982). Many of these patients might be dealt with on a day basis rather than an in-patient basis if suitable day facilities were available. At the very least the length of their in-patient admission could be drastically reduced (see pp. 70–2 for evidence of the feasibility of this). Similarly, a number of the already established long-term patients being followed up in the community will relapse from time to time and the question of admission to either an acute ward or a long-stay ward will be raised. Once again this picture of acute relapses in chronic conditions is an inherent feature of the course of chronic disabilities in the community (see pp. 20–1). Many of these 'acute-on-chronic' cases might also be dealt with on a day basis supported by the flexible use of back-up beds. Whether concerned with 'chronic-acute' cases, or 'acute-on-chronic' relapses, the day services can also act as a transition between in-patient and community status. Finally, day services offer the possibility of long-term maintenance care in the community with less of the disadvantages of long-stay care in hospital and possibly less of the expense. However, the temptation must be avoided to think that good quality care can be achieved without adequate resources (cf. Ch. 5).

We thus have a picture of what Douglas Bennett has called 'upside-down psychiatry'. In a traditional psychiatric service beds dominate and the day services are seen as an appendage, in a community-based service day places dominate and the beds are seen as an appendage (cf. the WHO report of 1953 in Ch. 2, p. 40). This requires a radical shift of attitudes. Can it be achieved? The answer to this depends upon our clarity of purpose and the resources made available. The DHSS guidelines for day care provisions are, day hospitals 0.3/1,000 of the population and day centres 0.6/1,000 (DHSS 1975). In 1976 Edwards and Carter found a shortfall of provision amounting to the equivalent of 100 day hospitals and 800 day centres, i.e. over 30,000 places (Edwards 1981). Given those kinds of shortages the prospects do not appear promising. It is also the case that these guidelines can themselves only be regarded as notional since, as Bennett (1981a) notes, it is doubtful if we can establish accurate policies and norms until we have better information and more reliable data concerning the limits and effectiveness of day services. He indicates that although the DHSS norms are in fact exceeded in Camberwell, nevertheless considerably more day services are still being planned. In general, day services are very much an under-used option and it is crucial that if care in the community is to become a reality for the long-term mentally ill then this situation must change.

It is likely that the main resource for such a change will have to be health authorities. As indicated, they have been the main providers up to now and with the financial stringencies currently facing local authorities, not to mention the lack of statutory obligations and specialized training to deal with the adult mentally ill, it seems inevitable that health authorities will have to continue to accept a large part of this responsibility in the future. This is not to say that there are not outstanding examples of local authority contributions to day services, e.g. the Worcester Development Project (Martin 1981) and contributions from the voluntary sector, notably MIND (Jowell 1981). Nevertheless, we have to look primarily to the health services. They have presided over the run-down of the mental hospital and they should therefore be presiding over the run-up of community services. In addition, these services should be specifically aimed at that client group (the long-term mentally ill) who have been most affected by the reduction in beds. The health authorities have a moral, as well as a statutory, responsibility to provide care. So, what do these day services need to provide? To quote Douglas Bennett again, the concept of a day hospital is of, 'a non-residential facility which will provide on a daily basis every, or almost every, form of treatment which could be provided on an in-patient basis' (Bennett 1976). Thus, we can now return to Bachrach's analysis of the manifest and latent functions of the mental hospital and examine the extent to which these can be met in day services.

## Long-term care

We noted earlier from Edwards and Carter's work that there is some evidence to suggest this is already happening in day services, particularly in day centres. As indicated, day care has a long-term support and maintenance function as well as the more acute, treatment and transitional functions. This is an important point to recognize as there is often a temptation to see day services in the context of a short-term, acute 'treatment', model. From all that has been said so far, this model has only limited application to the long-term mentally ill. Their needs for psychological and social support will not disappear any more than their needs for physical and material support. A comprehensive, community-based rehabilitation service will need to accept this. Of course, long-term support need not necessarily only be provided by day *hospitals* (although inevitably some patients will tend to stick in day hospitals and be difficult to discharge). Long term support may also be provided in other day units, e.g. day centres, sheltered workshops, social centres, etc. if such resources are available. But there are good reasons for wishing to mix the acute, transitional and maintenance patients as much as possible. Heterogeneity tends to benefit the most disadvantaged while not adversely affecting the care of the less disabled (see pp. 90–1). Thus, by being caught up in an active treatment milieu, the most difficult, chronic cases stand a better chance of being actively maintained and not lapsing into passive custodial care. They also stand a better chance of not being deprived of their fair share of resources (e.g. staffing).

## Asylum

Day care offers the possiblity of a partial asylum which is equally beneficial to the patient and his family and less harmful than the total asylum of the mental hospital. Thus, studies of schizophrenic patients in the community have indicated the possible benefits for some patients of reducing their face to face contact with highly critical or overprotective relatives (Vaughn and Leff 1976). Day care is one method of achieving this. Similarly, a day setting provides a more tolerant social environment, sheltered from the rigours and demands of life in the 'normal' world, while at the same time allowing the client to remain in contact with that world, for example by travelling to and from the unit each day. (This is actually a good reason for siting day hospitals away from the mental hospital as much as possible, something which had been done only in about a quarter of the units studied by Edwards and Carter (1979.) As well as providing asylum for the patients, day care can also provide relief for relatives. The studies to be reviewed later show very clearly that patients can be cared for on a day basis with no difference in reported family burden than if the patient had gone into hospital (see pp. 70–7). These studies also suggest that there are considerable advantages to the patient (even to his family) in terms of preserving role functioning to be gained by avoiding, or at least minimizing, admission. As described by Miles (1981: 106–14) the process of admission often leads to a progressive loss of social roles, the patient no longer participates in the household, and can no longer work, act fully as a parent, spouse, etc. However, when attempts are made to reduce or eliminate admission, social role functioning is far less severely disrupted. Thus, the patient is enabled to resume the ordinary activities and responsibilities of their lives very much more quickly.

## Accommodation

Obviously, the one thing that day care cannot do is provide accommodation. However, it can provide direct help with the everyday problems of living in the community, as well as assessment of, and training for, deficits in community living skills. In many ways day settings are particularly well placed to offer this kind of help, indeed much better placed than mental hospitals, since they do not suffer from the remoteness and artificiality of the hospital setting. Research on techniques of psychological assessment suggests very strongly that one of the major problems leading to a lack of validity in formal psychological tests is their 'specificity' (Mischel 1968). In other words, the tests produce results which are only specific to a particular situation and not necessarily representative of the person's functioning as a whole. One way of getting around this is to try to make the assessment setting as much like the criterion situation as possible. Thus, reducing the artificiality of assessment settings increases their validity. Hence, in a day setting one can observe the patient's problems in everyday living directly and then all you need is a simple check list with good content validity to make the assessment (Shepherd 1983a). In a similar vein, most psychological skills training programmes suffer from problems in generalizing, or transferring, the improvements from one setting to another (Shepherd 1980). Again, this 'generalization problem' may be minimized by making the treatment situation as much like the criterion situation as possible. Hence, if a person has problems in managing their money, using a launderette, going to the shops, travelling on a bus, etc. these are much better dealt with by working in those situations directly in the community, rather than from a hospital base.

## Medical treatment

As we have seen, the long-term mentally ill have significant needs for medical care both physical and psychiatric. Indeed, there are some reasons to suppose that their psychiatric needs may be even greater than those of long-stay patients in hospital since their conditions are less stable and they are more directly exposed to life-events (cf. Ch. 1, p. 5). In addition, many will be maintained on long-acting phenothiazines administered by injection and, given the possibility of harmful side-effects, the action of these drugs must be carefully monitored. There are thus strong reasons for wishing to ensure an adequate medical input to day services and this will be further reinforced if day settings are asked to undertake a more 'acute' treatment role. The care of the long-term mentally ill is *not* simply a social problem and this must be acknowledged by all those concerned (not least the doctors).

## Social and vocational help

As with the assessment and treatment of difficulties in everyday living, social and vocational problems may be directly assessed and treated with less of the difficulties of specificity and generalization inherent in a hospital situation. Day hospitals are well placed to undertake this initial assessment and treatment function providing they are given the right kinds of facilities and staffing (see Shepherd 1981a). As indicated above, they may need to pass on the longer term maintenance function in these areas to more specialized community-based facilities, e.g. day centres, sheltered workshops, social centres, etc. (The issues surrounding long-term social supports will be discussed at some length later in this chapter, see 'Families and Social Supports'; and the problems of vocational rehabilitation will be addressed in Ch. 6.) But the cornerstone of high quality care is an individually-centred approach (see Shepherd 1981a and Ch. 4) and this is particularly relevant when considering the questions of social and vocational help. Some patients will have greater vocational needs than others. For example, the typical middle-aged women with recurrent depressive episodes may benefit greatly from a fairly social atmosphere with an emphasis on everyday domestic tasks and simple social contact. In contrast, the young schizophrenic man may benefit more from help with vocational assessment and preparation in order to be able to return to work, or go on to retraining, or a sheltered workshop. These different needs should be reflected by the different activities available in day programmes and Edwards (1981) notes how little evidence there was of matching activities to individual needs. The programmes seemed dominated by simple social activities (record sessions, table tennis, card games) and there was little use of industrial or domestic work (Edwards and Carter 1979: 46–7). Unless day settings have a range of activities which offer adequate opportunites for normal role performance they cannot be expected to be able to counteract the influence of the 'sick role'. The more therapy-oriented the setting is, the greater this danger becomes. Of course, the balance of different activities may need to be modified slightly from 'normal' life. After all the clients are supposed to be 'patients' and some input of therapy is obviously necessary. However, the therapy can be fitted in around domestic or work activities, rather than the other way around.

*Custody*

The extent to which a day setting can provide a secure environment for psychiatric patients with criminal problems is obviously limited. However, day services can certainly assist in the transition of individuals from high

security settings back to more open community place-
ments, providing appropriate supervision is available.

## A comprehensive service

Day services should be seen as only one element – albeit
a crucially important one – in a comprehensive pattern of
psychiatric services. They are an alternative to beds, but
not a substitute (Bennett 1981a). In organizational terms
they can be seen as fitting in to the 'back door' of the acute
admission wards and before the 'front door' of the long-
stay wards. Thus, they not only attempt to interrupt the
circle of repeated admissions for the long-term patient on
the admission wards, they also, hopefully, reduce the flow
of new patients into long-stay beds. The extent to which
day services can perform this acute treatment function is,
as yet, unclear. The studies to be discussed later do
suggest that many patients currently dealt with on an in-
patient basis could be managed without admission with no
loss in effectiveness in controlling symptoms (e.g. Fenton
et al. 1982) and so the limits of day care are still relatively
unexplored territory. Given the need for long-term maintenance in addition to the more acute treatment, it might
seem sensible to conceive of day hospitals as a kind of
'clearing house' for major psychiatric illnesses. Assessments of individuals can usually be accomplished on a day
basis and treatment programmes begun, the clients may
then be referred on to other agencies for longer term
support if necessary. This would give a mix of the acute
and chronic day cases which was mentioned as desirable
earlier. A service of this kind does exist in the Camberwell
district (Bennett 1978c, 1981b) and as we shall see later
there is evidence to suggest that it has been both comprehensive and efficient.

## Employment

Day services offer secure employment for mental health
professionals. While it may be possible to care for long-
term patients more efficiently from a community base as

opposed to a hospital, there is no reason to suppose that the long-term mentally ill are going to vanish. There will be plenty of work to do although, as Bennett (1981a) notes, staff will require education and training to cope with these new ways of working.

Let us now move on to consider some of the other elements in a comprehensive community-based service.

## Accommodation

Traditionally, accommodation has come first in many people's minds when they have thought of alternatives to the mental hospital. But, as indicated earlier, there is a lot more to rehabilitation than simple resettlement outside hospital. In the future we need to put much more emphasis on day services and on preventing admission, as opposed to providing alternatives to hospital after the damage of a long admission has already been done. However, a range of options in terms of sheltered accommodation will be important and we should examine the needs of the various categories of long-term patient.

First, the old long-stay population: one of the most popular options for this group in the past has been the 'Group Home' (Ryan 1979; Morris 1981). This involves the creation of an artificial 'family' of three to four people while in hospital and then the preparation and discharge of what one hopes will be a mutually supportive group. Group homes have been particularly effective with the old long-stay patients who have already spent many years living together in a mental hospital. Adequate assessment and preparation is essential as many of these older clients will have lost the necessary skills for independent living in a modern community. In addition to certain skills, the prospective candidates also require motivation. They must actually want to leave hospital and from previous research we know that this will not always be the case (Wing and Brown 1970; Mann and Cree 1976). Of course, neither skills nor motivation are sufficient in isolation.

To assess and prepare clients for group home living a

realistic assessment unit is required together with a simple, but comprehensive, checklist of community skills. The assessment unit should provide the opportunity to observe the clients' abilities to cope with as many of the everyday tasks of living as possible, e.g. managing money, paying bills, shopping, cooking, cleaning, gardening, etc. It follows from what was said earlier that this setting should be as realistic as possible so as to maximize the validity of the assessment. This may be a difficult task for hospitals to achieve where such simple things as separate billing for services, separate catering and laundry budgets, and so on, can cause severe administrative difficulties. However, it should be stressed that if one has never had the opportunity to observe how patients cope with such demands then one has no real basis for making predictions as to how they will manage in the community. A good assessment can therefore save a lot of time and trouble in the long run. The outcome of such assessments provides the basis for remedial training programmes to improve areas of skills where deficits are apparent. In some cases these will be successful, but problems of 'generalization' (see p. 52) and the chronicity of disabilities will often limit the progress that can be made. A degree of mutual help is also sometimes possible, but there are limits to this and often all that one can do is ensure that staff are alerted to the patients' problems and that adequate attention is paid to supervising them on discharge. Supervision in the community is a crucial element in the success of group home schemes and psychiatric nurses working in the community or volunteers should strive their utmost to maintain close links with the hospital, general practitioners, etc. Given the nature of the clientele, group homes are nearly always something of a precarious enterprise. The most common problems are that patients lapse into self-neglect or neglect of their new environment. Engagement in other community facilities, e.g. day care, is thus important to maintain contact and keep them going.

Group homes normally operate with no supervision on

the premises and therefore a fairly high level of skills and independence is required. As indicated, they also tend to work best with people who have already lived together for some time and enjoy the benefits of communal living. For those who are relatively independent but would prefer more privacy, then housing association schemes, council housing, or even independent flats or bedsitters are possibilities, although from Christie-Brown et al. (1977) survey the numbers of old long-stay patients able to use these kinds of facilities are probably small (less than 10% aged under 65). For the more disabled a higher degree of supervision will be required, for example as in Part III accommodation for the elderly, or long-stay hostels. The remainder are so disabled, physically as well as psychiatrically, that hospital would seem to be the only option.

What of the new long-stay population? Mann and Cree (1976) suggested that about a third of their sample would require further care in a hospital-type setting although about a half of these have thought likely to respond to treatment and rehabilitation in the future. The numbers of new long-stay patients accumulating obviously depend upon the quality of day services and sheltered accommodation available locally. Nevertheless, in any service some patients will accrue who can only be cared for adequately in a hospital-type setting. A new kind of residential accommodation to meet the needs of this new long-stay group has been described recently by Bennett (1980) and Wykes (1982). It is a 'ward-in-a-house', or 'hostel-ward', and is organized around intensive individual nursing and psychological management programmes (see Lewis 1981). It caters for the most severely disabled patients and it may be hoped that small units of this kind will eventually replace the old long-stay wards of the mental hospital. In-patient beds are unlikely ever to disappear entirely from a psychiatric service, but a small number of acute beds together with a small number of this kind of highly specialized long-term places may be all that is required.

We can turn now to the long-term patient in the

community. Once again a variety of options are possible depending on individual needs and preferences. One of the most popular has been various sorts of hostel provision such as those described by Hewett et al. (1975), Ryan and Hewett (1976) and Ryan (1979). There are basically two kinds of hostel provision, short-stay and long-stay. The short-stay provision is conventionally envisaged as a stepping-stone between hospital and the community or between family and independent living. Short-stay hostels were very popular in the early days of attempts to empty the mental hospital, but as more severely disabled clients have been encountered, both in the hospital and in the community, so the impetus behind them has been somewhat dented. Short-stay hostels have been provided by a few hospitals, by local authorities, but particularly by voluntary bodies such as the Richmond Fellowship and the SOS Society. As more difficult clients have accumulated so the distinction between short and long-stay hostels has sometimes become blurred. However, as Ryan (1979) notes the latter are meant to provide more or less permanent sheltered accommodation for those long-term patients who are severely disabled and whose capacity for independent living is correspondingly limited. Long-stay hostels have been provided by local authorities and also by some voluntary bodies, notably the Mental After Care Association. There is a shortage of hostel provision according to the DHSS guidelines of 4–6 places per 100,000 (short-stay) and 15–24 per 100,000 (long-stay) and Ryan (1979: 60) estimates that in 1975 this shortfall amounted to over half the recommended places.

Although the characteristics of the short and long-stay hostel populations do differ somewhat there is a considerable degree of overlap, the most striking characteristic being the degree of social withdrawal observed in both groups (cf. Ch. 1, p. 12). They tend to have little contact with the other residents, few hobbies or leisure activities, few contacts with relatives and few social supports outside. They thus have little actual contact with the 'community' (they also tend to be unemployed and uninvolved with other day services. There is therefore a danger with hostel provisions of recreating long-stay wards in the community (cf. Lamb 1979) and, because many of these clients are so difficult and apparently unmotivated, extra attempts need to be made to involve them as much as possible in daytime social and work activities. On the other hand, one must guard against pushing one's own standards of social contact on to patients who may, quite rightly, discern their own need to withdraw. The line between over- and under-stimulation is always a difficult one to draw (see p. 68 below).

Other kinds of sheltered accommodation are described by Murray (1978) and Morris (1981) and these include hotels, guest houses, 'boarding-out' schemes (placement with selected landladies) and adult fostering. Leach (1979) and Leach and Wing (1980) also describe provisions for those who are totally destitute. All these services, including group homes and hostels, share certain problems in common. Firstly, the lessons of history (cf. Ch. 2) suggest that we must ensure adequate standards of care are maintained in both statutory and voluntary provisions. This is a considerable task, but some system of public accountability is the only mechanism that has ever been devised and attempts must continually be made to monitor standards of care (cf. Ch. 4). Residential care is also always expensive and those providing care must have adequate resources. Thirdly, there should be regular reviews of individual progress. As indicated earlier, this is the cornerstone of good practice and we need therefore to be able to distinguish very clearly between different levels of disability in terms of accommodation needs. These can then be met by the 'minimum therapeutic dose' of support required (Birley 1974), hence the need for a range of options emphasized by Wing and Olsen (1979). The problem with long-term care in the mental hospital is that it supplied the *maximum* 'dose' irrespective of individual need and this was one of the factors contributing to a loss of independent living skills. In order to facilitate such individually-centred care and review Ryan (1979) suggests local co-ordinating committees comprised of representatives from hospitals, local authorities and voluntary bodies involved in providing accommodation. There is certainly a need for co-ordination, but there is also a danger in this kind of arrangement in appearing to devolve this responsibility on to a single, small group of senior managers. As with other aspects of community services (e.g. day care) the best kind of co-ordination comes from the staff involved in the individual units having as much contact with one another as possible and hence a working knowledge of what is offered by other facilities. This is more difficult to achieve, but it helps reduce isolation and, by widening the information net, it makes referral and decision-making less vulnerable to breakdown through the absence of a single individual. Finally, as we have seen, sheltered accommodation needs to accept the presence of certain relatively fixed disabilities. Just as it is important to have some kind of system for identifying clients who may be improving (or deteriorating) and therefore require a different kind of care, so it is also important to accept some clients who are just standing still. With long-term psychiatric disability, maintenance is always a reasonable goal. Thus, some short-stay hostels may need to accept a longer term caring role than they might have envisaged. But, as Wing and Olsen (1979: 175) note 'if this is the highest level achievable . . . (then) . . . this is a form of success and not a form of failure'.

Of course, there is one other source of accommodation for the long-term patient – his family. As Bennett (1978b) has commented, families are nearly always available and – at least initially – they are often well motivated, they know the patient well, they speak his language, they rarely go on strike or ask for overtime and they can muster more beds than the National Health Service ever will. Yet, mental health professionals have generally not tried to work with this facility. How could they? What are the problems facing families and what kinds of help can the services offer?

## Families and social supports

In recent times psychiatry has neglected the families of the long-term mentally ill. This is a curious omission as we have seen how important they have been historically (see Ch. 2). Where families have been involved it has tended to be as the targets of abuse and criticism rather than as a valuable resource to be cultivated. The anti-psychiatry movement (Laing, Esterson, Cooper et al.) brought considerable distress, and largely unjustified blame, on to the relatives of psychiatric patients and we are only just beginning to move away from this polarized position. Although there has been considerable research (Jacob 1975; Neale and Oltmanns 1980) very little can actually be said with any degree of certainty regarding the aetiological significance of family factors in major mental illnesses. We can say that there is an *interaction* between certain family processes and the course of established psychiatric conditions. We can also speculate that this interaction extends back into the period before clinical symptoms are actually present. But this is a very different matter from having clear, specific, aetiological evidence. We cannot say that family processes 'cause' psychiatric illness any more than we can say the reverse. (Equally, the observed family interactions and the psychiatric symptoms might be unrelated causally and both produced by some unidentified third variable, e.g. social class, physiological arousal, etc., although this seems unlikely.)

The fact that there is a clear interaction justifies our being interested in the way that families affect patients and vice versa and this is especially important in a community-based service. When we become involved in community care for the mentally ill we inevitably become involved in working with families. Thus, patients may spend 40 hours a week in a day programme, but they will spend 128 hours a week at home. From the patient's point of view, if we can intervene to influence or reduce the adverse effects of family interaction then we might hope to improve and maintain functioning more effectively. From the relative's point of view, if we can make the patient's symptoms more tolerable we can at least reduce a part of their burden and they may then be more willing to care for the patient in the longer term.

We saw in Chapter 1 how it is common for long-stay patients to become estranged from their families and natural social supports in the community. This was undoubtedly due partly to a pattern of services which isolated patients in large, remote hospitals, making it difficult for families to sustain contact and leading to a closure of social roles for the patient. If, by providing local, community-based services we can treat patients more in their families, and at the same time offer these families adequate support, then we have the possibility of preventing long admissions and reducing some of the need for specialized sheltered accommodation (group homes, hostels, etc.). Obviously this will not be possible, nor even desirable, in every case, but residential accommodation of any kind is always expensive and we should be examining continually the most efficient ways of spending money. Perhaps if more were spent on supporting families, both directly and indirectly, this would be more cost effective. Prevention, where it is possible, is sometimes cheaper as well as better than cure.

The effects of family processes on the course of established psychiatric conditions have been described by Leff (1978) and Kuipers (1979). These studies began from an observation by Brown (1959) that schizophrenic patients being discharged from hospital to marital and parental homes seemed to have a worse outcome than those discharged to living alone or in a hostel. It was only those patients returning to homes where the family atmospheres were rated as showing high levels of expressed emotion (EE), particularly over-involvement and criticism who were at an enhanced risk of relapse. 'Over-involvement' refers to over-protective or over-concerned behaviour out of proportion to the realistic needs; 'criticism' refers to high levels of derogatory or disapproving remarks, usually related to something that the relative felt had always been a part of the patient's behaviour and that they always disliked. Patients returning to high EE homes had between three to four times the risk of symptomatic relapse within nine months (58% vs. 16%) compared with those returning to low EE homes (Brown et al. 1962, 1972; Vaughn and Leff 1976). In later studies it was shown that even within the high EE homes patients were at a lower risk of relapse if (a) they took regular medication (25% vs. 78%) and (b) they had less than 35 hours per week total face-to-face contact with their relatives (29% vs. 57%). In the most recent study these findings have been extended to include depressive patients. This research is very important and the general finding of a relationship between high EE and relapse has now received at least four independent replications. The implications of these findings for care and management will be discussed in a moment.

We can now turn to the effects that patients have on their families; once again this has been most extensively studied with regard to schizophrenia. Wing and Creer (1980) describe the results of a survey conducted with relatives who where members of the National Schizophrenia Fellowship. This study was mentioned in Chapter 1 (p. 12) in connection with the social withdrawal of long-term patients in the community and it was this feature that relatives reported most frequently (74%). They described the patients as taciturn, uncommunicative and making little conversation. They also reported how patients would withdraw from social contact, both within the family and with visitors and how they seemed to find just being with people an intolerable strain. The second most frequent kind of problem reported by the relatives concerned the patients' general underactivity (56%) and lack of leisure interests (50%). Relatives found it difficult to cope with the patients' solitary, seemingly rather barren, lives devoid of people or hobbies and often involving a great deal of sleeping. 'Slowness' was also quite often considered a problem (48%). Interestingly, socially embarrassing behaviour, self-neglect and poor meal-time behaviour were relatively infrequently reported, suggesting that these patients maintained a number of their very basic life skills quite well. Threats or violence and sexually unusual behaviour, although obviously upsetting if they occurred even once, were again relatively infrequent.

These relatives may not be typical of the relatives of schizophrenics in general, and schizophrenics are not the only category of long-term patients in the community (although they probably account for over a third). Nevertheless, the findings present a fairly coherent picture. Relatives complain of the social difficulties of living with psychiatric patients. They expect companionship and some social support and they are confronted with silence and withdrawal. They expect that this might be compensated for by increased interest in hobbies and leisure interests and yet apparently it is not. Under these circumstances perhaps it isn't surprising that relatives often begin to feel there must be something 'wrong' with them and anxiety, guilt, depression and anger are all common reactions. Because the patients' behaviour is often also unpredictable, relatives become frustrated. As one said, 'You just never know what he's going to be like from one hour to the next' (Wing and Creer 1980: 51). This creates a tense, awkward atmosphere and the patient withdraws further, making the situation worse, and so on. The mechanisms in the families of other kinds of long-term patients are no doubt somewhat different, but social withdrawal is also a common feature of depression and the relationship between high levels of criticism and relapse holds also for depression (Vaughn and Leff 1976). In depression one speculates that the patient's need for social contact is more straightforward and that it is his/her failure to obtain the right kind of supportive emotional contact that exacerbates their problems (cf. Brown and Harris 1978). Perhaps in depression it is more the case that relatives withdraw from the patient, rather than the other way around. But, in both instances the effect of these problems may be to isolate the family and reduce its contact with other relatives and friends outside. A similar phenomenon has been observed in families where one member is diagnosed as neurotic, see Collins et al. (1971). This further throws the family in on itself, further compounding the problems.

What help can be offered? In relation to schizophrenia the implications are clear: first, regular medication seems important. It significantly reduces the risk of relapse, even in the high risk homes. Presumably it somehow 'buffers' the patient against stress and allows them to lead a slightly more normal life. Secondly, simple reduction of face-to-face contact with high EE relatives further reduces the risk of relapse and the burden on families, hence the importance of day and other community services. It should be noted that staff will have to maintain an 'aggressive delivery system' (Davis et al. 1972) i.e. work hard, to ensure that erratic and unmotivated patients are actually involved in such services. Third, there is the possibility of some kind of 'family therapy' to examine whether any of the mismatches between expectations and performance can be resolved, or if some of the longstanding roots of critical comments can be explored. Family therapy is a complex area and there are considerably more theories than facts (see McPeak 1979; Walrond-Skinner 1981). However, some attempts have been made to work with the families of long-term patients and perhaps effective techniques will be developed (e.g. Glick and Kessler 1980; Falloon et al. 1981). At the very least, if community-based services can be persuaded to adopt a 'family approach' (Bennett et al. 1976) then some progress might be made.

A family approach simply consists of working with the families right from the outset, offering them information and involving them in the care and management of the patients' problems. In the case of schizophrenia this involves offering them basic information concerning what is known about schizophrenia, its origins, symptoms, course, the importance of medication, etc. Families often complain that they are told nothing about their relative's condition and as Kuipers (1979) notes this may sometimes be due to a genuine failure on the part of the professionals involved who themselves often feel at a loss. Families need information concerning the services available (financial, supportive, voluntary, etc.), where to go when problems arise, how to mobilize their general practitioners, who to contact at the hospital, etc. They also need advice on management, what to expect, what to ignore, how much to protect the patient, etc. This is obviously the most difficult area and several attempts have been made to involve families in self-help groups (e.g. Priestley 1979; Ekdawi 1981) so that they might learn from one another.

One of the most important principles to emerge from studying how families cope with a condition like schizophrenia seems to be the value of maintaining some kind of 'distance' from the problems. Once relatives become embroiled in emotional confrontations difficulties can quickly ensue, however if they can separate practical from emotional issues and maintain certain basic expectations, while also remaining sympathetic, this seems to be the most effective strategy. This often depends on making a judgement as to what is due to the 'illness' and what is not – a difficult task – and, as was commented in Chapter 2, perhaps relatives should be encouraged sometimes not to feel that it is always a necessary decision to have to make. 'Can't?' or 'Won't?', perhaps it doesn't really matter, the problem is still there and it has to be dealt with somehow. Kuipers (1979) lists a number of useful management strategies for coping with schizophrenia at home, and these include: (1) set clear rules and standards; (2) coax sympathetically, but don't pressure; (3) know when to ignore; (4) don't argue with delusions, accept their subjective reality while not necessarily agreeing with their objective truth; (5) use distractions and (6) use humour (occasionally). For schizophrenics, the central problem is probably the tightrope between over- and under-stimulation (cf. pp. 58–60) and as we saw earlier this applies equally to those in hostels as it does in families.

Regarding other categories of long-term patient, advice on management is harder, since it is less clear whether any general problems can be identified. However, from the research cited earlier with minor depressive illnesses (Brown and Harris 1978) some similar principles seem to apply. For example, the importance of supportive social contact, the need to negotiate clear patterns of expectations within the home, and the importance of contacts and activities outside it. For all long-term patients, families deserve to be involved in discussions about how their relatives' management in the community is to be handled. For example, when admissions to hospital are going to be necessary, why and for how long, when admissions to day care programmes are appropriate and what the aims are. Unless we are prepared genuinely to work with families in the business of community care, we run a considerable risk that they will work against us.

All this implies a considerable involvement of staff and part of the problem, as indicated, is that there is often a lack of professional expertise. This cannot be filled by a single professional group, e.g. psychiatric social workers. A 'family approach' (as opposed to 'family therapy') does not necessarily require great sophistication, it simply implies a willingness to talk to families and to try to enlist their help and co-operation. At the very least it implies a willingness to listen to their complaints – often a highly under-rated skill. These are not complicated demands. One would hope therefore that all staff might be involved in a family approach: all psychiatric nurses not just community psychiatric nurses, all doctors not just the specialized family therapists. Families are untrained and unqualified but are expected to cope, why should the professionals be embarrassed? Staff, however inexperienced, can at least offer a reliable, sympathetic ear and perhaps more than anything else that is often what is most needed.

As for other social supports, we have already emphasized the importance of day programmes and it is worth remembering that, particularly for Social Classess IV and V, the main sources of friendship and social contact are still work and the family (Young and Wilmott 1975). Other informal, drop-in social centres have been described (e.g., Brandon 1981; Wilder 1981) and these can offer opportunities for social contact on a controllable, 'non-threatening' basis. They can also offer a comfortable warm place to go and cheap food, all of which may be invaluable to individuals who are materially, as well as socially, deprived. The concept of social supports and social networks will be discussed more fully in Chapter 6, but let us end this examination of care in the community by looking at the most important question of all: 'will it work'?

## Effectiveness and efficiency

Cochrane (1971) makes a fundamental distinction between 'effectiveness' and 'efficiency' in the evaluation of health services. He suggests that we use the term 'effectiveness' to refer to the demonstration of the effects of a particular procedure within a research context, particularly the random controlled trial. Conversely, he suggests that we use the term 'efficiency' to refer to the results obtained when the procedure is applied in routine clinical practice in a defined community. The procedures that we have been concerned with in this chapter, those involved in providing a community-based service for the long-term mentally ill, may be evaluated from both these perspectives. Because community care is an approach, not a single 'thing', it cannot be evaluated by a single trial. It requires a number of controlled trials of different aspects of the approach and also the collection of evidence as to how the total approach affects the psychiatric morbidity and use of services within a given population. This can only be supplied by epidemiological data, i.e. data concerning the distribution, course and outcome of disorders. We shall review both types of evidence here. The aim is not to provide proof that community care has been a 'success', that would be an unrealistic task (like trying to prove that education had been a success) but simply to point to some examples of research-based effectiveness and at least one example of what seems to be a reasonably efficient service. More extensive reviews are to be found in Test and Stein (1978), Wing (1978c) and Fenton et al. (1982). So, first we will consider research-based effectiveness. All these studies compare conventional policies of hospital admission with various kinds of community-based alternatives.

Glick and Hargreaves (1979) compared short (i.e. 3–4 weeks) vs. long (i.e. 8–16 weeks) admissions to hospital and their effects on a group of schizophrenic patients and on a second group with mixed diagnoses (affective disorders, neuroses and personality disorders). All the patients were initially admitted to hospital and then randomly assigned to either the 'short' ($n = 117$) or 'long' ($n = 118$) admission group. Few patients were omitted from the study and the only exclusions were those who: (a) left too early to be evaluated satisfactorily; (b) were not aged between 16–45; (c) had IQs less than 70; (d) were alcoholic, epileptic, addicted to drugs, or with serious physical illnesses. Despite randomization, within the schizophrenic sample ($n = 141$) the 'long' admission group had slightly better early educational backgrounds and social adjustment. In the 'short' admission group planning for discharge was begun immediately, there was a clinical and social assessment and treatment goals were formulated aimed at resolving practical living problems and providing symptom relief. Long-term recommendations were made, usually for further treatment or rehabilitation measures to be pursued after discharge. In the long admission group a generally similar policy was implemented although without the pressure on time. Staff used the longer admissions to attempt to prepare the patients for involvement in subsequent after-care facilities (e.g. vocational retraining, out-patient visits). All patients were assessed using a variety of reliable and well standardized measures of clinical, social and vocational functioning. Families were also asked to evaluate the patients' condition. Ratings were made on admission, after four weeks, on discharge and at one and two year follow-up.

The results indicate that in the schizophrenic group the short admission patients improved rapidly and by the time of their discharge were functioning much better than their counterparts in the long admission group. However, by the time this group were ready for discharge they had equalled or surpassed their colleagues in the short admission group. Over the follow-up period, the long admission group appeared to fare slightly better, although this was partly explicable by their good premorbid adjustment (these patients were over-represented in this group to start with). The authors attribute the better long term outcome for the long admission schizophrenic group to better involvement with out-patient services and better compliance with medication. For the non-schizophrenic group the results were more straightforward. In short-term admission patients pulled together more quickly and the long-term patients gradually caught them up such that there were no differences over the follow-up period. The authors conclude that the demands of a short admission mobilize staff, patients and relatives to cope more quickly with a rapid return to the community. They note that there may be some reason to extend admissions for the schizophrenics with a good prognosis as this seems to engage them more effectively in after-care services, but there is no reason to extend admissions for the more chronic schizophrenics, or for most of the non-schizophrenic disorders. (They acknowledge the possibility that for some of the affective disorders a longer admission might sometimes be useful to assess suicide risk more adequately.) In terms of rehospitalization in the follow-up period there were no differences between any of the groups. This study therefore casts doubt over the policy of long admissions (say more than four weeks) for most long-term patients, particularly chronic schizophrenics. With more intensive work with families and in the community might this be cut down even further?

Fenton et al. (1982) studied a more acute group of patients and compared treatment given in hospital with similar treatment given while they remained out of hospital and at home. The patients were a mixed group of schizophrenics (40%), manic depressives (29%) and depressive neuroses (30%). The majority had at least one previous psychiatric admission. All patients were initially assessed in the 'emergency room' of a general hospital and referred on for possible inclusion in the study if they were thought to be in need of immediate admission. A number were then excluded (almost half) if they were considered to be too great a suicide risk, or if they were suffering from some kind of organic condition which required investigation in hospital. A further third then had to be excluded because they presented on a day or at a time when the research team could not complete the initial interviews. This left about a fifth of the original number who were then randomly assigned either to treatment based on hospital ($n = 79$) or to treatment based at home ($n = 76$). In both cases this relied fairly heavily on psychotropic medication, with simple counselling and practical help of various kinds given by multi-disciplinary team. For the home-based group this centred around meetings with the family (or friends) and social casework of a problem-solving kind. In-patient admissions were kept to an absolute minimum. For the hospital-based group the treatment was given by a standard clinical team who looked after the patient in hospital for as long as they thought necessary and then provided follow-up in the community after discharge. All patients and their relatives were assessed at the outset and after 1, 3, 6 and 12 months by independent assessors once again using a range of reliable and standardized measures.

The results were clear-cut: viz. (1) The home-based treatment was just as effective in controlling symptomatology as the hospital-based treatment. (2) There were no differences with regard to the reported burden on the families between the two groups. Indeed there was some evidence of decreased burden in the home-based group resulting from the fact that the patients were still able to cope with some of their domestic responsibilities even though they remained psychiatrically impaired. (3) Some deficits in role functioning persisted in both groups, particularly among the schizophrenics. For example, patients who were unemployed before the illness episode were likely to remain unemployed after it. (4) Some family problems, e.g. financial difficulties, also persisted in both groups even after the disappearance of symptoms. (5) The home-based programme was considerably cheaper to run, mainly because of the reduced use of in-patient admission (on average over the whole year, 14.5 days vs. 41.7 days). This study therefore suggests that with a relatively acute population, lengths of admission may be cut quite dramatically provided adequate help is given to the patients and their families in the community. Further-more, this need not result in an intolerable burden being placed on the families or on other community services. The authors are at pains to point out the limitations of their existing community facilities (Fenton et al. 1982: 91) and speculate that more extensive services would: (a) improve the effectiveness of the service (op. cit.: 119) and (b) extend its capacity to deal with more disabled clients (op. cit.: 125).

Some of these possibilities were examined in a study by Test and Stein (1978) comparing a community-based treat-ment programme ('Training in Community Living') with traditional hospital admission for a mixed group of adult patients all of whom were originally seeking admission. The patients were relatively young (mean age: 31 years) but had spent on average 12–16 months in psychiatric hospitals before the study began. The only exclusions were: (a) not resident locally; (b) not aged between 18–62, and (c) severe organic brain syndrome or primary alcoholism. The patients were assessed by the admissions staff and then randomly assigned to either community-based treatment ($n = 65$) or hospital-based treatment ($n = 65$). The community treatment lasted fourteen months and consisted of intensive support and direct help with various problems of everyday living. A group of typical mental hospital ward staff (nurse, psychiatrist, psychologist, occupational therapist, social worker) were retained to provide daily, even hourly, assistance to individual clients. Help was given concerning independent living skills, i.e. washing, cooking, laundry, etc., also assistance in finding a job or sheltered workshop placement and extra support when this was first started. Patients were 'prodded' to involve themselves in relevant community recreation and social activities and make more constructive use of their leisure time. Families were contacted and meetings held to discuss progress and 'constructive separation' if necessary. All the programmes were tailored to the needs of the individual client and admission to hospital was avoided wherever possible. (The programme is described in detail in Stein and Test 1978.) The hospital-based group were treated in hospital for as long as was deemed necessary and then linked with appropriate community agencies. All patients were assessed from the beginning and at 4-monthly intervals for 12 months using a battery of clinical and social instruments. Self-reported satisfaction with life and self-esteem were also measured and families were interviewed where available to assess family burden (about a quarter of the sample).

In clinical terms the results indicated that the community-based treatment group generally showed less symptoms throughout the period of the study. In social terms, they spent less time unemployed, earned more, had more 'contacts with trusted friends' and belonged to, or attended, more social groups. There were no differences regarding other leisure-time activities and social contacts. The community treatment group reported great overall satisfaction with their lives and had higher self-esteem from the outset. There were no differences in reported family burden. Over the 12 month period the community group spent on average 2 days in hospital compared with 29 days for the hospital group. A complex cost-benefit analysis indicated that while the community treatment programme involved larger direct costs (largely due to staffing) it involved smaller costs in every other form (indirect treatment, low enforcement, maintenance, family burdens). Considering all forms of cost in total, the hospital programme was about 10 per cent cheaper (Weisbrod et al. 1980). These findings sound a note of caution to those who might hope that care in the community is necessarily care 'on the cheap'. Although the quality of functioning achieved may be superior, it is not always less expensive. The authors also note that early observations of patients' performance since the programme has stopped suggest that some deterioration in functioning was beginning to take place. They comment that 'Training in Community Living' needs to be an ongoing, permanently available service if chronic disability is to be prevented.

Finally, there are some studies directly involving day care. Herz and his colleagues have reported a series of papers comparing day and in-patient care. In the first of these, Herz et al. (1971) screened newly admitted acute in-patients to determine whether day treatment could be used as an alternative to their admission. Approximately one third were rejected as being too suicidal, violent or disorganized. Another 20 per cent were considered too well. This left ninety patients who were considered suitable (50% of whom were schizophrenic). They were then randomly assigned to day or in-patient care. There was an initial assessment and assessments at 3 months, and up to 3 years follow-up. Clinical state was examined and various aspects of role functioning. The results indicated that the day hospital group showed slightly quicker improvement in their clinical symptoms over the first month, and over the follow-up period more improvement on scales evaluating 'Daily Routine', 'Leisure Time Impairment' and

'Housekeeping Role'. The day hospital group spent much less time in hospital and their readmission rate was half that of the hospital group over a 9 month period.

In the second study Herz et al. (1975, 1976) compared standard in-patient care with a brief in-patient admission followed by referral to day-care or out-patient care. A mixed group of newly admitted in-patients were included ($n = 175$), 63 per cent were schizophrenic and slightly over a half came from Social Classes IV and V. The only important exclusions were alcoholics, drug addicts or personality disorders. Patients were assessed at 3 weeks, then again at 3, 6, 12, 18, and 24 months. Clinical symptoms and social role functioning were rated using standardized measures and families were interviewed. At 3 and 12 weeks there were no differences in clinical symptoms between any of the groups, all had improved substantially. This was interesting because, as the authors note, substantially less medication was used in the Brief groups compared with the Standard group. As would be expected social role functioning was much less impaired in the Brief groups (despite their symptoms) as these patients were able to resume their roles very much more quickly. There were no differences in reported family burden except at the very beginning (after 3 weeks) when the Brief groups did report some increase in difficulties. Throughout the study, families showed signs of worry, anxiety and distress irrespective of the treatment modality of their relatives. Also, 28 per cent of *all* families believed the patient had been sent home to soon (including the Standard group). In fact the average lengths of stay were 11 days for the Brief groups and 60 days for the Standard group. Over the follow-up period the Brief groups continued to be hospitalized less and show less social impairment (Herz et al. 1977). The authors conclude that their studies clearly indicate the value of brief admissions followed by day care support for the majority of acutely ill psychiatric patients. They suggest that such a policy should be cost-effective.

All the studies reviewed in this section suffer from methodological flaws. Although reliable and standardized measures have been used, together with independent raters, the possibility of some influence of 'experimenter bias' has to be acknowledged. This is almost impossible to eradicate completely. There are also variable rates of attrition from a number of the samples, but again this is virtually inevitable in research conducted in service settings. Overall, the studies constitute an impressive body of evidence. They suggest very strongly that a policy of care in the community with short admissions can be effective for very many psychiatric patients. There seem to be no significant disadvantages in terms of controlling symptoms with significant advantages with regard to reducing social role impairments. All this can be achieved without unacceptable burdens being placed on the family or other community resources and probably without great expense. However, can such services be maintained? Can they work efficiently over prolonged periods of time?

To answer these questions we need to consider some epidemiological evidence. One community-based service which has been studied in some detail is that of Camberwell (Bennett 1978c, 1981b; Wing and Hailey 1972; Wing 1978c). In 1964 Camberwell had a traditional psychiatric service in which patients with a recent illness and good prognosis were admitted to a university teaching hospital (the Maudsley) while those who needed readmission or were chronically disabled went to mental hospitals, mainly Cane Hill situated fifteen miles away. The service was developed in an essentially pragmatic fashion with the aim of decreasing or containing psychiatric disability for the patient, his family and the community at large. It was not the policy to concentrate on discharge, but rather to provide services which were local and which gave the patients the help they needed without admission (Bennett 1976c: 274). This was achieved by expanding day hospital and local authority day centre provisions and other support services, for example, a Resettlement Workshop, sheltered factory, Housing Association, 'drop-in' social support, etc. In this way care was gradually moved from being centred upon the hospital to being centred upon other units and services. The mental hospital remained as a back-up service to be used when needed, but it no longer dominated. A new District Services Centre (Bennett 1981b: 166) has recently opened providing extensive day-care facilities and some of its own in-patient beds.

These changes have been documented by the Camberwell Case Register (Wing and Hailey 1972) which is a data-linkage system for collecting and reporting information about all Camberwell residents who suffer from mental illness or mental retardation and who are in contact with the psychiatric services. The Register data reveal a gradual decrease in the numbers of old long-stay patients, mainly through death rather than discharge, and a steady accumulation of new long-stay and long-term patients in the community. About two-thirds of the new long-stay patients are over 65 years of age. A new specialized residential unit has recently been opened for the younger patients and this was described earlier (see p. 58). The new long-term patients are dispersed through the community in a day hospital, day centres, or with their families. The day hospital (now the District Services Centre) acts as a focus for these community-based services. Thus, although admission rates have not changed substantially overall (neither have they nationally, MIND 1980) the locus of care has gradually been successfully shifted from the mental hospital towards more community-based alternatives, particularly day-care. Bennett (1978c: 288) acknowledges that the Register data does not tell us whether these alternatives have actually offered a better *quality* of care, however the controlled trials cited earlier suggest that this is likely to be the case.

Care in the community for the long-term mentally ill therefore can be a reality, and we have some reason to believe that it can be made to 'work'. But shifting the locus of care from the hospital towards the community is not a sufficient change in itself to eradicate psychiatric disability. We somehow need to ensure that a high quality of care is maintained irrespective of the treatment setting. How this might be accomplished will be addressed in the next chapter.

## Summary

Maurice Chevalier was reported to have responded to the question, 'How do you like growing old?' with the reply, 'Well, not very much, but I prefer it to the alternative!' Perhaps that is an appropriate verdict on community care at the present time. It is by no means perfect, but it appears preferable to the alternative. We have some understanding of the medical and social functions that hospital care served and provided we take care to ensure that services are created in the community which, as far as possible, replace these functions then the patients should not suffer. Indeed, they might even benefit. Day care provides the key to these services, it gives an institutional base in the community from which many of the services previously offered by the hospital may be located. Day services together with a range of back-up resources, including beds, thus constitute the core provisions of community care. A community-based service is also immediately a family service. Working with the families on the problems of the non-daytime hours becomes just as important as working with the patients on the problems of the daytime hours. There is also enough evidence now, both from random-controlled trials and epidemiological data, to suppose that these developments might lead to a pattern of services for the long-term mentally ill which is both effective and efficient.

# Chapter 4

# Quality of care

'Quality of Care' is a difficult concept. This is partly because it is not definable by a single measurement operation. It is also partly because nobody is quite sure what should be subsumed under its heading. What variables determine a high 'quality of care'? What reasons do we have to suppose that these variables will exert an influence on patients' functioning and what are these effects likely to be? These are the questions to be addressed in this chapter.

We begin with the assumption that 'quality of care' is a composite, rather than a single, variable. Thus, it is similar to the concept of institutional 'ethos' introduced by Michael Rutter and his colleagues in their study of secondary schools in Inner London (Rutter et al. 1979). They were interested in discovering whether schools *per se* had an effect on pupils' attainments and behaviour irrespective of the composition of the original intakes. They found evidence of such an effect and they labelled this the 'ethos', or institutional 'climate', of the school. It was composed of a number of separate factors (e.g. the degree of academic emphasis, teacher action in lessons, availability of incentives and rewards, good conditions for pupils, extent to which the children were able to take responsibility, etc., see op. cit.: 178), however, their combined effect was more powerful than that of any individual factor considered on its own. We assume that an analogous composite variable – 'construct' would be a more psychological word – exists which defines 'quality of care'. We further assume that such a construct may be applied to any setting which provides long-term care and that this may be done irrespective of whether it is a long-stay ward in a hospital, a day hospital, or even a family home. 'Quality of care' is thus characteristic of how the setting operates, not where it is located. What variables does it consist of?

## Size, staffing and physical facilities

We saw in Chapter 2 how one of the factors leading to a deterioration of standards of care in the new asylums was their rapid increase in size and consequent overcrowding (p. 35). 'Small is beautiful' (Schumacher 1973) is a fashionable slogan, but is there really a straightforward relationship between size and quality of institutional care? Bella (1976) has reviewed the evidence on this topic in relation to residential care for the mentally handicapped and concludes that, although care was generally more adequate in smaller institutions, there was still considerable variation. He noted that there was very little evidence to suggest that the behavioural functioning of residents was different in institutions of different sizes. There were essentially no data on the issue of whether smaller institutions were more adequate than larger ones in terms of returning their residents to the community, but there was a little evidence to suggest that parental and community involvement might be enhanced in the smaller facilities. Thus, whatever the relationship between size and quality of care, it is not a simple one.

Further light is shed on this issue by the work of Raynes and her colleagues (Raynes et al. 1979). She suggests that certain organizational factors are characteristic of large-scale facilities and it is these factors that we need to isolate in order to understand how size *per se* relates to standards of care. These factors will be discussed in some detail below (see 'Organization and Management Practices') but one of the most important ones seems to be the size of the smallest autonomous management unit. Thus, it is not the overall size of the institution that is important, but the size of the units within it that have control over their own operation. A large institution can therefore offer a 'non-institutional' quality of care, providing it allows its internal units some degree of autonomy. (N.B. This factor, as with the others that we shall be discussing, should not be seen as exerting its influence in isolation. There is a cumulative effect, and the management autonomy of small units is a necessary, *but not sufficient*, condition for a high 'quality of care'.) In terms of specific size, Raynes et al. (1974) argue that living units of more than thirty clients will have difficulty in sustaining resident-centred, and therefore high quality, care.

A similar complex interaction emerges when we consider staffing. Obviously, below a certain minimum level of staffing a high quality of care is not possible. Sutton (1981) suggests that the staffing ratio in the current DHSS guidelines of one trained nurse to three patients is insufficient to carry out active rehabilitation programmes and yet this is often still not met. However, above a certain minimum level, the addition of extra numbers is no guarantee that standards of care will improve in proportion. It then depends upon how staff are organized and what they actually do. King et al. (1971) found no relationship between crude staffing ratios and quality of care, although all the units they studied had reasonable staffing levels. However, there were differences in *effective* staffing ratios. For example, the practice of allocating maximum staff to living units at peak periods (meal-times, bedtime, etc.) was associated, although not strongly, with a more resident-centred style of care. Conversely, where staff were allocated with no regard to peak and slack periods, standards of care were generally poorer. Similarly, Lewis (1981) stresses the importance of nursing staff being organized such that they can work intensively with small groups of patients (8–10) and accompany them through the different physical locations and activities of the working day. In this way individualized plans of care are more likely to emerge. Stability of staffing may also sometimes be more important than simple numbers. For example, Hall and Baker (1972) have described the problems in setting up a Token Economy regime where the staff were continually being moved on to their units. Thus, allocation, organization and stability are all potentially important factors, in addition to total numbers of staff, in determining the quality of care that will be offered.

As far as the physical facilities required, these have already been mentioned earlier (see Chapter, 1 pp. 18–19 and Chapter 3, pp. 51–4). Essentially, they consist of providing opportunities for normal social and role performance, i.e. realistic settings where the normal activities of living, working and social interaction can take place. Without these there is the danger of what Miller and Gwynne (1972) have referred to as 'social death' occurring. They studied residential institutions for the physically handicapped and young chronic sick and noted that, 'to the extent that patients are seen to be incapable of occupying any role that is positively valued by society, they are in effect socially dead' (op. cit.: 9). They went on to argue for the use of work and work substitutes as a way of importing normal role relationship into institutional settings (op. cit.: 151–3, cf. also 'Work' in Ch. 6). We saw in Chapter 3 how community-based care can also open up a wider range of opportunities for normal role performance.

Psychologists working within a behaviourist perspective have similarly emphasized the importance of the environment in eliciting and maintaining adaptive behaviour (see, for example, Whatmore et al. 1975). They argue that the environment should always be arranged such that adaptive behaviour is elicited and reinforced, and non-adaptive behaviour is extinguished. Thus, nothing should be done for the patients which they can already do for themselves. This simple dictum flies in the face of many of the basic assumptions of hospitals and of the sick role. All too often patients' skills and abilities are allowed to deteriorate by providing *more* care than they actually need. Even a simple feature like the seating arrangements can have a direct effect on functioning. Thus, Keddie (1978) has shown how different physical patterns of arranging chairs have significant effects on social interaction and the amount of active and passive behaviour in a psychiatric day room. These are the basic resources and facilities, but what of how such settings should actually be organized and run?

## Organization and management practices

The most vivid pictures of institutional practices in modern times have been given to us by Goffman (1961). We saw on p. 46 how he described the 'total institution' as breaking down the barriers which ordinarily separate the activities of sleep, work and leisure. Community care helps break up the 'total institution' by locating these basic activities in geographically separate places, but this is not enough. We must also consider the organization and management practices *within* each unit. Goffman (1961: 17) went on to describe these in the 'total institution':

> First, all aspects of life are conducted in the same place and under the same single authority. Second, each phase of the member's daily activity is carried on in the immediate company of a large batch of others, all of whom are treated alike and required to do the same things together. Third, all phases of the day's activities are tightly scheduled, with one activity leading at a pre-arranged time into the next, the whole sequence of activities being imposed from above by a system of explicit formal rulings and a body of officials. Finally, the various enforced activities are brought together into a single rational plan purportedly designed to fulfil the official aims of the institution.

Goffman's style was formidable, but his methods were impressionistic and it was not until some years later that an attempt was made to operationalize his ideas and to translate them into more formal, scientific terms. The late Jack Tizard and his colleagues began a series of studies on institutional care for severely mentally handicapped children which have been mentioned earlier (see King et al. 1971). They developed a number of rating scales to identify four main dimensions of management practice:

1. *Rigidity of routine*. The extent to which the residents conformed to an inflexible timetable of events. Did they all get up at the same time? Eat at the same time? Go to work (or activities) at the same time?

2. *Block treatment*. The extent to which residents were cared for 'en masse' as opposed to singly, according to individual needs and abilities. Was everybody given the same activity? Were there individual care plans?

3. *Depersonalization*. The extent to which residents were given personal possessions and private space. Did they have their own clothes? Toiletries? Recreational materials?

4. *Staff – patient 'distance'*. The extent to which staff maintained clear divisions between themselves and the residents. Did they wear uniforms? Eat with the clients? Were there separate toilet facilities? A staff 'lounge'?

They then used these scales to evaluate a number of residential settings. Each setting was rated on a number of items relating to each of the main dimensions and a score assigned according to whether the management practices seemed to be 'institutionally-oriented' or 'client-oriented'. The former referred to those practices which seemed to exist mainly to serve the needs of a smooth running organization, the latter referred to those practices which seemed to exist to meet the needs of individual clients. They found a considerable variation in the organization of the different homes, however it was possible to identify two extreme groups corresponding to either end of the institution vs. client dimension. The research team then entered these units and performed a number of direct observation studies on the amount, nature and quality of the staff-child interactions.

This revealed some striking findings. The staff in the 'client-oriented' units were observed to interact with the children significantly more than the staff in the 'institutionally-oriented' units. Furthermore, they tended to interact more warmly, and in a way that was labelled as more accepting and less rejecting. There was also less difference between senior and junior staff members in terms of their responsibilities and the amount of contact they had with the children in the 'client-oriented' homes. These differences were not attributable to the severity of the handicaps of the children, nor to the size of the units, nor to the staffing ratios. However, they did seem associated with staff training and backgrounds, in addition to the management practices outlined above. These results have subsequently been replicated in local authority day centres for the adult mentally ill by Shepherd and Richardson (1979a).

What these studies demonstrate is a consistent picture of organization and management practices reflected in the amount and nature of staff-client interactions. How the units were run and what happened in them thus appeared to be reflections of a single process. This raises some intriguing questions of causal interpretation and these will be discussed later (see, 'Causes and Effects'). However, for the moment we shall focus on the implications for organization and management practices. If we assume that a 'non-institutional' style of care is desirable, then it seems that certain features must be present in the organization of care settings in order that it will be possible for such a style of care to develop.

First, individually-centred management programmes must form the cornerstone. (This also implies some flexibility of routines.) We saw in Chapter 2 how the importance of individual care was emphasized by the early pioneers of institutional care and how this was gradually eroded by various social and political pressures. The need to 'treat patients as individuals' is a familiar theme, but there may often be little evidence of it in practice. Edwards (1981) noted how little matching there was between activites and personal needs in many day care settings and unfortunately this is often the case both in hospital and in the community. It is often associated with an over-emphasis on group treatments. Of course, there is nothing wrong with group treatments providing they are arrived at as part of a programme specifically designed to meet each individual's needs, but too often they are part of a blanket prescription which everybody gets irrespective of their actual needs. Individually-centred programmes can also come into conflict with a medical/treatment orientation. Thus, it may be difficult to conceive of an individual adapting at different levels in different areas of disability (e.g. work and living) if one is operating with a fixed, global notion of 'cure'. The concept of cure implies only two states: 'well' and 'ill', and it is then difficult to conceive of an individual being 'well' enough to manage living independently, but too 'ill' to be able to find a job in open employment, or vice versa. Individually-centred patterns of care also require fairly intensive staff-client interactions and hence the importance of staff allocation, organization and stability mentioned earlier. King et al. showed that one reason why there was more equality in the amount of client contact between the senior and junior staff in the more resident-oriented units was that senior staff in the institutionally-oriented units had less freedom to delegate their administrative duties. Where senior staff had more choice over how they would organize their time, they delegated more and spent more time with the children. This is an example of the complex interactions between resources, organization and staff-client interaction and we shall have more to say about this later.

After individually-centred management programmes, we come next to the question of patient autonomy.

Patients need to be given the opportunity to take certain decisions for themselves. For example, what clothes they will wear, when to shave, when to go to the bathroom, when to have a cup of tea, etc. They also need to be able to exercise choices within a framework of expectations determined by others. For example, whether they will eat at a particular time cr go without, whether they will go to work or stay in bed, etc. These are choices we all have to take and they are a fundamental feature of normal social roles (cf. Ch. 1, pp. 16–17). To deprive patients of such choices is to deprive them of a part of their identity as people. As Miller and Gwynne (1972: 19) put it, 'Institutional life reinforced their dependence in a way that deprived them of the rights and obligations of other adults to make quite ordinary decisions about their own lives'. Of course, the 'normalizing' value of providing opportunities to take decisions lies in striking the correct balance between personal autonomy and working within the expectations of others. But, patient autonomy should not be the *only* ingredient involved in care. Settings which over-emphasize personal autonomy do not prepare clients to accommodate to other people. Conversely, settings which over-emphasize external expectations allow no room for personal expression and fulfilment. (This may have been a part of what happened in institutions following the triumph of legalism over medicine, cf. Ch. 2, pp. 34–5.)

The reduction of staff-patient 'distance' is perhaps the most straightforward of the implications for creating non-institutional styles of care. At a personal level, the research on the effectiveness of psychotherapy suggests very strongly that therapists who are able to be open and honest with their clients and not hide behind professional façades are likely to be the most effective (Truax and Carkhuff 1967; Beck et al. 1979). Counselling is a central part of the rehabilitation process (Ekdawi 1981) and the skills involved are therefore very important to foster. In physical terms, the physical separation between staff and clients should also not be too rigid. For example, Sanson-Fisher et al. (1979) reported evidence of marked 'territories' for staff and patients in an in-patient psychiatric unit attached to a general teaching hospital. They found that on 85 per cent of the occasions that patients were observed they were in specific 'patient areas' of the ward (mainly their own bedrooms), on only 3.6 per cent of observations they were seen to be in 'staff areas'. Conversely, staff were observed to be in their own areas on 56 per cent of occasions, but also in patient areas on 28 per cent of occasions. Thus, patients appear to remain within their own 'territories' much more than staff do. This is not surprising given the nature of staffs' responsibilities but, as the authors note, this physical segregation reduces the possibilities for patients to engage in therapeutic interactions with staff. The more sharply these physical lines of demarcation are drawn the less possibilities for interaction there are. (In this study staff believed that they should spend at least 50% of their time in those areas where patients spend the majority of their time, in fact they only spend 28%.) The wearing of uniforms is another potential physical barrier between staff and patients, but unfortunately there seems to be little research on the issue of how staff clothing affects the levels and quality of their interactions.

Before we go on to consider staff-client interaction in more detail, we will consider one other important organizational variable. In general terms there seems to be an inverse relationship between chronicity of handicap and allocation of resources, i.e. the most chronically disabled get the least resources and the least chronically disabled get the most. This seems to be connected with the higher status and priority given to 'treatment' as opposed 'care'. Thus, 33 per cent of all beds in the National Health Service are in mental illness and mental handicap hospitals, but they account for only 13 per cent of the total expenditure. Similarly, costs per in-patient week are two to three times as much in acute services compared with mental illness or mental handicap (MIND 1980). We therefore have a situation where 'ghettos' of long-term disability are created in long-stay wards or institutions which are unattractive to both staff and resources. How can these be prevented?

Adequate allocation of resources is obviously one factor, but as we have seen it is not the whole story. There are more complex processes at work. One method through which the effects of these concentrations of disability may be ameliorated is to have some mixing of levels of handicap. Although King et al. found no relationship between level of handicap and quality of care, theirs was a relatively homogeneous sample. In a larger survey of over 20,000 patients from 79 programmes in 34 hospitals throughout North America, Ellsworth et al. (1979) report that the major finding was that patients who were admitted and treated on wards in which there was a mixture of acutes and chronics had a better outcome in terms of community adjustment after two years, than those treated on wards with more narrowly defined selection criteria. They note that their results clearly support the rationale for an 'unclassified unit system' and warn against the dangers of a drift towards wards filled with chronically hospitalized patients.

Obviously, there may be limits to which such mixing of patients is possible, for example, it may not be desirable to group psychiatric with physical patients, or acute patients with psychogeriatrics. Nevertheless, hetero-geneity *within* client group seems to be an important principle. It helps maintain staff morale since they are not continually being confronted with 'failure' and apparent lack of progress. It also helps to avoid segregated care and the separation of 'first-class' patients who receive all the 'treatment' from the 'second-class' patients who receive only 'care'. The greatest benefits are potentially for those who are most disabled and it is unlikely that those with less severe disabilities will suffer. In any event their prognosis is generally much better. It seems again that there may be a parallel here with education, as Rutter et al. (1979: 202) comment upon the considerable disadvantages of an educational system which allows a markedly uneven distribution of intakes with a heavy preponderance of the intellectually less able. Mixing levels of disability may sometimes come into conflict with a desire for specialization and this is a difficult problem. Where allocation of resources, staff morale, etc. can be maintained in specialized units they are obviously useful; but in practice this often seems difficult to achieve. Mixing 'acute' and 'chronic' admissions seems a better general safeguard for maintaining high standards of care for all. We turn now to the problems of staff-client interactions.

## Staff-client interaction

Rehabilitation may not require great technical sophistication, however it does depend upon the frequent and high quality interactions between staff, or other carers, and the clients. The first point is therefore to ensure that adequate levels of staff-client contact do occur. Unfortunately, in many long-stay wards this is often not the case. Even in more acute settings, levels of staff-patient contact can be quite low. For example, in the study by Sanson-Fisher et al. (1979) mentioned earlier staff spent only 23 per cent of their time interacting with the patients whereas they spent 41 per cent of their time interacting with colleagues. Conversely, patients spent 78 per cent of their interaction time with other patients and only 22 per cent with members of staff (op. cit.: 322–4). These kinds of findings suggest that perhaps we should not be concentrating on staff-client interaction at all, but on client-client as this seems to be the more significant. Nevertheless, staff-client interaction is usually considered the main vehicle for therapeutic change, so how should staff be using their contacts with their clients to the best effect?

The mechanisms underlying effective therapeutic interaction with long-term patients are controversial. A wide range of approaches has been tried from the behavioural (such as token economies) to 'milieu therapy' (such as therapeutic communities). They have met with varying degrees of success but most approaches can claim to have some demonstrable value. Indeed, Erickson (1975: 528) concludes after a lengthy review of different treatment programmes in hospital with the rather wry comment that: 'it is tempting to conclude that practically any reasonable innovation will lead to improvement'. While this may be going a bit far, the similarities in outcome do lead one to speculate that different therapeutic approaches might have a lot more in common when it comes to explaining the process of change than might appear from their superficially very different theoretical rationales (Shepherd 1980). What might these common ingredients be?

This question is easiest to answer by drawing on the research with token economies, which have been shown to be effective with the most disabled long-term patients (Paul and Lentz 1977). In a series of studies Hall and Baker found that staff expectations, feedback on performance and social approval were just as important as the physical administration of a token in maintaining the improvements of long-term patients (Baker et al. 1974, 1977; Hall et al. 1977). The generality of these findings is still in some dispute and Elliot et al. (1979) have suggested that tokens *per se* may be crucial to effect change, although they may not be necessary to maintain improvement. Nevertheless, the factors of expectancy, feedback and social attention do seem widely applicable. They are prominent features of 'milieu therapies' (Gunderson 1980) and seem plausible candidates as common underlying mechanisms of treatment. Thus, if staff maintain high (but realistic) expectations, if they can communicate these to the patients with clear and specific feedback, if they do this reasonably contingently and with a measure of sensitivity and social approval, then the outcome should be that patient functioning is effectively improved and that the improvement is maintained. This does not seem too far a cry from the 'Christianity and common-sense' of the moral treatment era (cf. Ch. 2, p. 31). Nor does it seem substantially different from the methods employed by relatives who cope well with schizophrenic patients at home (cf. Kuipers 1979, Ch. 3, pp. 67–8). It also echoes the judicious mixture of firmness and warmth favoured by Sinclair (1975) as the ideal combination for residential care staff in Probation Hostels. These ingredients therefore do seem to be fundamental, so what kinds of staff are likely to display them? And, can staff be trained to do so?

King et al. (1971) found a significant association between institutional training and the tendency to operate institutionally-oriented patterns of care. Similarly, Shepherd and Richardson (1979a) found a direct correlation between staff attitudes to management practices and the quality of staff-client interactions. Thus, there is evidence to suggest that staff training and attitudes affect the quality of their interactions with clients. Staff should therefore be given careful training and direct feedback on their performance with patients. This can be achieved in a number of ways. Classroom teaching is an obvious approach, but other methods are required if actual behaviour on the ward is to be affected. For example, staff groups in which attitudes and behaviour can be examined with peer group support (cf. 'Maintenance and Support', pp. 94–7). Alternatively, a system of close monitoring and feedback on individual patient's progress can help staff to organize and structure their interactions more effectively (Lewis 1981). This feature has been suggested by Hall et al. (1977) to be one of the major reasons why token economy regimes are liked by staff and why they are successful.

Of course, not all staff will make effective therapists and this fact has to be acknowledged. Their skills can be used in other ways, but we must always try to ensure that those who do bear the brunt of the direct contact with clients are not always the most junior and lowest status members of the team. They should receive the same support and recognition for the contribution as the high status, 'hit-and-run', professionals (e.g. psychologists, doctors, social workers, etc.). If they do not, then a vital element in maintaining a high quality of care will be lost. It must also be acknowledged that not all staff can be trained to be effective therapists. This is not an argument against training, but we do need to recognize that good methods of selection are often just as important as sophisticated packages of training.

The outcome studies also demonstrate that few treatment programmes show an appreciable effect on clients' functioning for long after they have left the immediate setting (Shepherd 1980). Thus, an active, therapeutic approach to care has to be maintained over long periods. How can this be achieved?

## Maintenance and support

Maintaining a high quality of care is rather like maintaining an antiseptic environment. It is not a battle that is ever won once and for all, instead it is a continuing struggle against infection. The sources of infection in this case are lack of resources, overcrowding, institutionally-oriented management practices, ghettos of concentrated disability, low levels and poor quality of staff-client interaction, etc. can these be counteracted?

This is a matter for senior managers and administrators, those who are involved in planning and providing the service must provide the necessary back-ups and support. These can take many forms. First, as we have seen, the direct-care staff are often the most junior people and they require both technical and emotional support. In the same way as the relatives of schizophrenics (cf. Ch. 3, pp. 66–7), they need to be given information about who they are dealing with, what the likely outcomes are, what facilities are available, advice on management, and so on. All this comes under the general heading of staff training and education. Perhaps more importantly they also need direct support at work. For example, the reassurance that they are doing the 'right thing', someone to complain to about just how difficult their job undoubtedly is, etc. Senior managers can also help to set the right kind of institutional 'ethos' by involving staff in taking decisions as to practices and policies within the unit. Norma Raynes' most recent research emphasizes perceived involvement in decision-making as the most important single organizational variable contributing to client-centred patterns of care (Raynes et al. 1979). This can be achieved through regular weekly unit meetings where staff have the opportunity to support one another in dealing with the inevitable conflicts and crises, and can also discuss important matters of policy and practice. The involvement of senior managers in these meetings is crucial. To return to the educational parallel, Rutter et al. (1979: 193) note the importance of a prevailing consensus on the values and aims of the school as a whole and the importance of all staff being involved in the formulation of this.

A second method through which senior staff can help maintain standards of care is by fostering good teamwork. Since psychiatric rehabilitation depends upon people, not technology, the successful management of direct-care staff is crucial. Watts and Bennett (1983) have recently reviewed some of the literature relating to these management issues from a social psychological point of view and they emphasize the importance of involvement and consent if decisions are actually to be carried out. 'No implementation without participation', seems a good general rule. They also stress the necessity to share information and argue against the use of 'key workers' on the grounds that a single individual is unlikely either to be adequately informed, or adequately available, to meet the necessary demands. The importance of 'good communication' may be a cliché, but unfortunately it is a true one. Watts and Bennett also discuss the question of leadership and point out the need for senior managers to establish credibility by demonstrating a commitment and a willingness to be involved in the day to day work of the unit (even if it is only in terms of regularly attending one meeting a week). They draw upon the psychological research relating to the qualities of effective leaders and emphasize that providing social supports is just as important as providing clarity and problem-solving skills. Finally, they discuss the question of conflict resolution and note that conflicts are an inevitable (indeed a healthy) part of teamwork. The leader's role should be to use conflicts to arrive at good compromise solutions which embrace different points of view and improve cohesiveness rather than damaging it. Good teamwork is about motivating staff and, although it may not be possible to conjure up motivation if none is there in the first place, it is certainly easy to destroy it through careless and insensitive management.

A final method through which staff may be supported and quality of care maintained is by the provision of change and innovation. Again, we saw in Chapter 2 that a part of the reason for the decline in institutional care was the disillusionment that set in as a result of the accumulation of apparently intractable cases. We may detect here again the pervasive influence of models of care based upon treatment and 'cure', but it is understandable that staff need to feel they are making some progress and that their efforts are not being wasted. There are a number of ways in which this need can be met. First, staff must be aware of the nature of the disabilities that they are dealing with (cf. Ch. 1). When one is faced with a declining baseline, just to be 'standing still' is often a considerable achievement. Second, staff can be helped to focus upon their achievements, however small, in improving and maintaining functioning. Setting clear, specific and limited goals and reviewing progress is not only good practice from the patients' point of view, it is also crucial in keeping staff motivated. Clear information and feedback are just as potent in changing staff behaviour as they are in changing that of clients and perhaps the most important contribution of the behavioural approach has been its emphasis on identifying small and gradual changes. Thirdly, a conscious policy of introducing change and innovation can be adopted. The introduction of students can help and it will be facilitated by providing situations where staff come into regular contact and discuss among themselves policies and practices to be followed within the unit. Senior staff can also help by indicating a willingness to review traditional procedures. Another possibility, is the use of therapeutic 'holidays' for either staff or patients. For example, an intriguing study by Rezin et al. (1979) documents the gradual decline over time in staff-client interaction in a token economy and they suggest periodic breaks, or 'holidays', to counteract boredom and gradual loss of enthusiasm. This is not a mindless prescription of 'change for change's sake'. There are obvious limits, but the capacity to develop new ways of dealing with old problems represents the life-blood of any long-term care setting. When this is lost, the practice may become ossified and standards will begin to deteriorate. A high quality of care is essentially based upon an active and optimistic approach and this optimism must be clung to in the face of the most severe contradictions. If it is not to be lost entirely then some hope of change, if not for the patients, at least for the institution, must be continually kept alive.

All this relates to care staff and their work, however there may also be issues of a more personal psychological nature which affect staff. There are personal issues for any person in any job and sometimes these do affect his/her work. This is particularly true in the case of the sick and disabled. Isabel Menzies (1970) has written about the psychological problems for nursing staff in dealing with disease and death and the defences that these evoke. There is a case therefore for providing all staff with emotional support on a personal basis should this be required. Again, if senior staff make themselves clearly available for this function, they will then be used as necessary.

## Causes and effects

'Quality of Care', as we have seen, is a complex variable. It is composed of a number of factors at the level of physical resources and facilities, organizational practices, staff-client interactions and back-up supports. How are these related causally? Do certain physical features 'cause' certain management practices to arise which then determine particular kinds of staff-client interactions? Or, do certain kinds of staff support facilitate staff-client interaction which then gives rise to a particular style of management? Or is it the management practices that are the key factors? Or the degree of patient autonomy? Or the right kind of staff-client interaction? Or the right size? Or, in the end is it all a matter of staffing levels and resources? Put in this way the *naiveté* of expecting simple answers is clear. Psychiatry, particularly the history of long-term care, is replete with people who thought that they had found 'the answer' in everything from whirling patients round in chairs to leaving them to fester in their own excrement. Of course, there is no 'answer'. That is, there are many answers and the composite construct 'quality of care' discussed here attempts to summarize some of them. But, it is not clear just how important each individual element is and, as indicated at the beginning of this chapter, there are many necessary, but not sufficient, conditions. It is not even easy to sort out such effects through multivariate statistical methods (e.g. multiple regression) as the size of their individual contribution may be small. Their combined effects may also be different in different contexts. To cite Rutter et al. (1979: 183) again: 'the same teacher actions sometimes led to quite different results in different schools'. Thus, all that we can do is attempt to specify the factors which seem to be important and try to ensure that as many as possible of them are fulfilled.

Even if they are fulfilled, what are the effects likely to

be? What reasons, apart from humanitarian ones, do we have to suppose that a high 'quality of care' as defined here will actually benefit the patients? In the first place, we can cite some negative reasons. Many of the features described here such as the opportunities for normal role performance, individually-centred patterns of care, high staff-client contact with clear expectations and feedback, etc. were conspicuous by their absence from traditional institutional care and this was certainly associated with low levels of functioning (and 'institutionalism', see Wing and Brown 1970). However, this kind of argument is correlational, i.e. it relies on an association between the variables which tells us nothing about their causal interrelation. Certainly, it is clear that institutional practices did not 'cause' institutionalism in any straightforward sense. Institutionalism was the product of an interaction between certain features present in the patient's environment and certain predisposing factors present within the patients themselves (Paul 1969). However, there are also some positive reasons. Thus, it is clear from the research on token economies that a well organized staff, working with clear, individually-centred programmes, based on high levels and a good quality of staff-patient interaction, can effectively improve and maintain functioning (Paul and Lentz 1977). Hence, if such standards are maintained then functioning should be improved and maintained. The effectiveness of regimes like token economies does not sustain the case for all the factors that we have been discussing here, but it covers many of them. We thus have both positive and negative reasons for supposing that our construct of 'Quality of Care' may be important for patients, as well as for institutions.

In the last two chapters we have sketched out an alternative pattern of care for the long-term patient based on community services and on a particular view of what constitutes high quality of care. These ideas have implications for current services and the ways in which existing provisions need to be changed. How can such changes be brought about? This is the issue to be addressed in the next chapter.

## Summary

'Quality of Care' is a complex construct. It does not consist of a single factor or dimension, rather it is composed of a number of separate variables. These include size, staffing, physical facilities, organization and management practices, levels and quality of staff-client interaction and the adequacy of staff supports and back-up facilities. In general terms, the maintenance of a high standard of care seems to depend upon the provision of individually-centred management programmes which contain clear expectations and the opportunity to engage in normal social roles and where the clients receive praise and encouragement for their efforts within the context of a sympathetic relationship. To achieve this and maintain it for the most disabled some mixing of levels of disability (acute and chronic) seems desirable. Direct-care staff should also be involved as much as possible in taking management decisions concerning the operation of their own units and should be helped to work effectively as a team. Novelty and change seem important. The causal interrelationships between these variables at different levels in the system are complex and no single element should be given overriding significance. There are reasons, both positive and negative, to suppose that if such standards of care are met then this will have a beneficial effect on patients' functioning.

# Chapter 5

# Creating organizational change

Creating change in mental health services is an ambitious undertaking. In a classic paper Georgiades and Phillimore (1975) have described the tendency of large institutions to devour 'hero-innovators' just as dragons devour brave knights. However, these authors also provide some strategy guidelines to assist the managers of change and there are other relevant areas of psychological research which give some clues as to how change might be achieved. It is the purpose of this chapter to bring some of these ideas together and to provide some hints for would-be 'heroes'. Given the paucity of experimental evidence in this field, these ideas cannot be guaranteed as a proven recipe for getting your own way. Nor are they a potted handbook for political subversion. Nevertheless, perhaps they will provide a few words of caution, and just a little advice, for those who wish to stay at least one step ahead of the dragon.

A convenient framework for thinking about the problems of institutional change is provided in the general 'problem-solving model' described by D'Zurilla and Gold-fried (1971). These authors were interested to apply research findings from the problem-solving literature to behaviour modification with individual clients. However, the same model may also be applied to changing the function of institutions or the patterns of health services. The problem-solving model involves a number of stages, viz.: (1) Defining the Problem; (2) Considering Alternative Solutions; (3) Implementation, and (4) Feedback and Evaluation. Each of these will now be considered.

## Defining the problem

Georgiades and Phillimore suggest that to initiate a planned programme of change in hospitals or community settings the initiator must first consider very carefully the question 'Who is my client'? Mental health professionals are accustomed to defining their work in relation to the care of individual clients, however to create institutional change it is necessary to view the entire organization or health care system as the client. Thus, Bender (1979) has described the three possible levels of psychological intervention:

1. *Working directly with clients individually or in groups*.
2. *Working with staff*. Transmitting assessment or therapeutic skills and allowing them to deal directly with clients. (This is the so-called 'triadic intervention' model, see Tharp and Wetzel 1969.)
3. *Working with managers*. Those who formulate policy and allocate resources. These are the 'planners and providers' who tend to operate at a senior management level and remain fairly remote from actual direct contact with clients (cf. Ch. 4, p. 95).

Bender notes that psychologists should be prepared to operate at all these three levels; however, given the shortage of professional manpower (Hawks 1971) working through staff and working to create the right context for service delivery seem particularly important. But psychologists will have little credibility to work with staff and transmit technical skills (level 2) unless they have already demonstrated some degree of effectiveness in dealing with individual clients. Similarly, work at levels 1 and 2 will be undermined, or made effectively impossible, without adequate resources allocated at level 3 (cf. again Ch. 4,

p. 89). There are also strong arguments in favour of those who are responsible for planning a service being involved, at least minimally, in delivering it. This kind of management accountability should not be overlooked. So, in this chapter we will be particularly concerned with the processes at level 3 and the methods through which the right kind of climate for institutional change can be created.

If the health care 'system' is accepted as the appropriate target for change rather than the individual client, then how can we set about analysing the problem? This question has two kinds of answer: first, in terms of the change-agent (i.e. you) and second, in terms of the institutional context (i.e. other people). Defining the problem for yourself means understanding how the present system operates and understanding how—and—why you want to change it. Health services consist of three essential ingredients: places, patients and staff. Thus, the first task is to acquaint yourself with what facilities are available in your area, what their functions are and how they operate. It is essential in this exercise, especially in the current economic climate, not to restrict this survey to those facilities provided by the statutory services (Health and Local Authority). We saw in Chapter 3 how important the voluntary sector has been in relation to community-based care and this is likely to continue to be the case in the future. It is therefore essential that any aspiring change agent should know as much about the local non-statutory services as the major statutory providers. In any given community there are often many more of these non-statutory organizations operating than might be expected on first acquaintance (e.g. MIND, National Schizophrenia Fellowship, Mental After-Care Association, Church Army, etc). A useful start may simply be to ensure that these different bodies are actually aware of one another's existence. Regular, informal meetings (e.g. lunches), say once a month, may be a good way of achieving this. It is sometimes striking how, even in a small community, each different facility remains almost completely isolated from each other and this is often particularly true of the hospital and voluntary services. Comprehensive community-care will almost inevitably be based upon a 'patchwork' of services and getting to know each component and fostering communication between them is therefore a crucial first step.

Next, we come to an examination of how the patients move through this network of services. We need to find out why some get lost or 'dumped' at various points, why some find their way out at the other end but others leave after only one or two contacts (cf. Goldberg and Huxley's 'filter' model and the 'sluices' analogy in Ch. 1, pp. 3–4). If one is interested in changing the pattern of services one must first understand the variables that control these movements. For example, it is necessary to recognize the effects of severity of pathology – that only the most severely disabled progress further and further into the system. Similarly, those patients who come regularly into hospital and stay the longest tend to be those who are the poorest and who have the least social supports outside. These characteristics set them apart from other groups of patients in the 'system' and, although there may be some degree of overlap, each different category of client circulates around essentially separate pathways. (This idea has important implications for the prevention of long-term psychiatric disability, see Ch. 6.) When one has some understanding of how patients 'flow' through the system, one can then try to predict what effects changes in these pathways will have. For example, if day services begin to take new chronic patients early from the acute admission wards, then this should: (a) interrupt the cycle of repeated readmission and thus reduce the pressure on acute beds, and (b) reduce the rate of accumulation of new 'long-stay' patients and thus relieve some of the pressure on long-stay beds. Of course, all this will depend upon staff being able to identify the new long-term patients while they are still on the acute admission wards and on there being a good working relationship between the acute services and the longer term rehabilitation units. Hence, we now need to move on to the third ingredient in the system, the staff.

Decisions concerning movements (admissions, discharges, transfers) are obviously dependent on the staff involved. It is thus necessary to discover who takes these decisions and on what basis. Who are the 'gatekeepers' to the service and why and how do they decide that someone should be taken into hospital, referred for day care, placed in a group home, etc? Traditionally, the majority of events leading to admission to hospital involve the patient behaving in a way that is either a clear danger to themselves or others, or is markedly disturbed or abnormal, e.g. shouting, swearing, wandering about (Brown et al. 1966: 48). However, there may be considerable variation in the degree of disturbance tolerated by different staff members and, in general, staff will be more prepared to take a 'risky' decision (not admit, refer to day care rather than in-patient care, etc.) if they are given some kind of back-up or support (Kogan and Wallach 1967). Some decisions may also be taken on the basis of poor information or simple ignorance of the alternatives. Hence, it is important that staff are provided with adequate assessment instruments (checklists, etc.) and that they are informed of the range of options that are available (cf. p. 55). In terms of making more use of community-based services, one therefore needs to work with those key members of staff who control admissions and discharges and help them to think of community options rather than automatically reaching for a 'bed'. It should also not be assumed that admissions and discharges are always controlled by doctors. Doctors are often not available when patients are admitted, and may anyway be very much influenced by senior nursing staff (charge nurses and sisters). In day settings particularly, nursing staff often exert more or less complete control over who comes in and out. One must therefore acknowledge the importance of their contribution in determining the movement of patients. (It is a fact that the ratio of nursing staff to doctors in mental illness hospitals is approximately 15: 1, see MIND 1980.)

Having understood something of how the present system operates, the next task is to understand how you want to change it. It is good to begin with a very clear – and possibly somewhat grandiose – overall objective. For example, to close a particular mental hospital and replace it entirely with community-based services. The advantages of having a somewhat unrealistic aim to begin with is that you then always have unachieved goals to keep you going. Of course, you will also need some more realistic sub-goals to give a little reinforcement along the way. For example, the development of day services, the shift of resources from in-patient to community, the development of non-statutory support services in the community, etc. A clear objective and a clear ordering of priorities are therefore essential requirements for institutional change. It is the case that 'in the land of the blind, the one-eyed man is King' and even 'half an eye' can make you a perfectly reasonable Privy Councillor! One of the major reasons for needing clear goals and sub-goals is that they give yardsticks against which new developments may be evaluated. Inevitably, the change process will not go as you plan it and it is therefore necessary to have some method of evaluating which changes are useful and which are irrelevant, or possibly damaging, to your cause. For example, is the development of a separate Community Psychiatric Nursing Service a good or a bad thing as far as the rehabilitation of long-term patients is concerned? (Answer: it is probably a bad thing if it diverts resources away from long-term patients and towards primary health care.) Having clear goals and clear priorities thus enables you to *anticipate* the effects of change, your own and other people's. This ability to anticipate accurately the outcome of events is one of the hallmarks of intelligent activity. Thus, Douglas Bennett (1978c: 273–4) describes how it was necessary for himself and a consultant colleague to be given staff appointments in *both* an independent teaching hospital (Bethlem and Maudsley) and NHS hospitals (King's College and St Francis) in order to prevent patients from being cared for in remote mental hospitals and redirect them towards more local, community-based services. Their ability to anticipate events and to see how changes in their own service would effect, and dependent upon, changes in other services was a vital factor in their success.

Of course, clear goals and priorities have to come from somewhere and the experience of visiting, or better still working in, a different health care system that seems to be operating effectively is very useful. The change agent also needs some kind of personal motivation and his/her own value system is therefore important. Good reformers tend to have strong religious, humanitarian, or political values (unresolved Oedipal conflict is always a good standby). It should also be remembered that personal motivation can usually only be sustained with the help of others, and hence there is a need for group support (see 'Implementing Solutions' below).

So much for defining the problem for oneself, what about defining it for others? This is a time-consuming exercise. Institutions are composed of people and the most important mechanism through which institutional change occurs is therefore through a consensus that certain changes are necessary and desirable. Hence, persuading others to accept your definition of the problem and some of the goals and sub-goals necessary to remedy it may actually be the *sine qua non* for achieving change. Of course, this will often not be achieved without some change in your own views and your ideas will be modified through your interaction with others. But the first step is to raise people's awareness that problems exist and that they can be solved. This is rather like creating what the advertisers call 'brand-awareness' so if, for example, your product is better day services, then the first stage would

be to go around saying to everyone endlessly and mono-
tonously, that 'Day Care is a good thing'. At this stage it
is not even necessary to be particularly selective in who
you say this to, the aim is simply to implant the idea in as
many minds as possible. Catchy slogans may be useful in
this connection, for example, Douglas Bennett's 'upside-
down psychiatry' (p. 49). People are much more likely to
remember brief, discrete ideas than long, complicated
arguments. Once large numbers of staff begin talking
about a particular service development then it stands some
chance of being adopted, even if it has to be somewhat
altered in the process. If the ideas remain in only a few
people's heads, then the likelihood of widespread change
is correspondingly limited. The initiator should therefore
concentrate on 'preparing the culture' to accept change
and this will necessarily be a patient and slow business.
Georgiades and Phillimore (1975: 317) suggest that it
may be best to concentrate first on the 'healthy' parts of
the system, i.e. those that have the will and resources to
improve. Certainly, the initial aim must be to foster a
consensus of optimism that change is possible, indeed inevitable. If everybody starts talking as though some kind
of change is 'just around the corner' then something is
almost bound to happen.

## Considering alternative solutions

The next stage is to consider the alternative possibilities
for action. The key factor here is to involve as many
people as possible in the process while not sacrificing too
much of your original aims. (Hence, the importance of
having a clear initial understanding of your aims and
overall strategy; inevitably, tactics will have to be made
up as you go along.) Involving a number of people is
important for two reasons. First, the success of any change
will ultimately depend upon the goodwill and co-operation
of other people and we saw in Chapter 4 how staff are

much more likely to be willing to carry out decisions if they have been involved in formulating them, Second, there is some experimental research on decision-making which suggests that group 'brainstorming' techniques do facilitate the production of good quality alternatives in problem-solving exercises (D'Zurilla and Goldfried 1971: 114–17).

These brainstorming techniques depend on two basic principles: (a) deferment of judgement ('generate don't evaluate') and (b) quantity breeds quality ('the more the better'). There are therefore four basic rules.

1. *Criticism is ruled out*. The 'no criticism' rule seems to work particularly well in facilitating solutions to problems that subjects are already familiar with (as opposed to novel problems). It seems to help free them from the restrictions of previously held cognitive 'sets'.

2. *'Free-wheeling' is welcomed*. Subjects are encouraged to think freely, the wilder the idea the better. Original ideas seem to spark off associations which then lead to more and better ideas.

3. *Quantity is wanted*. This has received the clearest empirical support and indeed the notion of 'quantity breeding quality' is implicit in all the brainstorming rules. Interestingly, the research seems to suggest that the best ideas tend to appear later, rather than earlier, in the output.

4. *Combination and improvement are sought*. Subjects are encouraged to combine ideas or suggest how ideas might be improved. This is the least substantiated of the general rules in terms of experimental evidence; however, it seems intuitively plausible.

D'Zurilla and Goldfried note that it is not possible from the evidence to specify which of these four rules is the most important, thus they probably do not need to be all that strictly adhered to. Nevertheless, the principle of using groups to generate a range of alternative solutions is an important one. There is a crucial distinction to be made here between the usefulness of large groups to

generate ideas and to advise and consult and the usefulness of small groups to implement specific courses of
action. 'Consultation' and 'implementation' are two very
different management processes and, while it may be
effective to use a relatively large group of people to advise
and consult, this is not likely to be an effective way of
implementing decisions. Committees are not good at
writing letters.

We turn next to the process of selecting from among
alternatives the most suitable course of action. In the first
place, any proposed course of action should be clear and
specific. Thus, it should be capable of passing the 'Hey-
Dad, Watch-me-while-I' test. This means that it should be
sufficiently concrete for its occurrence or non-occurrence
to be clear to an independent observer. 'Arranging a
regular monthly meeting between the admission ward staff
and staff from the long-stay area', or, 'ensuring weekly
supervision of family work in a day centre by an experienced social worker' would both be actions that would
pass the *'Hey-Dad'* test. 'Improving communication with
the admission wards', or, 'making family work more
important in the day centre', are both examples of actions
that would not. (They are sometimes known as 'fuzzies'.)
In addition to being clear and specific, goals should also
be realistic and attainable. Since all change is likely to
encounter resistance, and the amount of resistance is
likely to be in direct proportion to the amount of change
involved, there are good reasons for choosing initial
courses of action that lead gradually towards the final
objective. Fairweather et al. (1974: 188) refer to this as
the 'Foot-in-the-Door' principle. There are also other
reasons for choosing 'piecemeal' rather than revolutionary
change. For example, gradual change offers the possibility
of learning from your mistakes, making them one at a time
rather than all at once. Small changes are also much more
likely to be achievable than large ones and successes –
however small – are the crucial elements necessary to
sustain the change agents. Finally, a strategy of gradual

change will often be forced upon you by circumstances. It simply isn't possible to change things quickly in large bureaucratic organizations and one may as well treat this necessity as a virtue and dwell upon the positive aspects of gradual change rather than the negative ones.

In the Fairweather et al. (1974) study just mentioned, a number of variables were found not to be related to organizational change and these are worth discussing. Their research was an ambitious project concerned with evaluating the effectiveness of different methods of persuading hospitals to set up a demonstrably effective 'lodge' programme (a kind of half-way house) for the rehabilitation of long-stay psychiatric patients. The authors studied the value of sending written manuals, conducting workshops and setting up live demonstrations and the project concerned over 200 mental hospitals throughout the United States. Each method was evaluated in terms of how effective it was in establishing these lodge facilities over a two-year period. Some of the variables that emerged as unrelated to adoption were the status, finance and resources of the hospitals involved. Thus, change was as likely in hospitals situated in traditionally 'conservative' parts of the country as in those in traditionally 'progressive' areas. The lack of a relationship with money was particularly striking. Fairweather et al. (1974: 183) comment that there is at best a questionable relationship between the allocation of resources and the effecting of tangible institutional change: 'You can pay for progress, but you can't buy it'. Thus, in terms of choosing a suitable initial course of action, perhaps one should not be put off by the fact that there is no money available (there never is). If the idea is a good one, and enough people support it, then money will be found. If the idea does not receive widespread support, then no amount of cash will ensure its implementation. There are certainly many examples in the rehabilitation field of considerable achievements being made by pioneering groups or individuals with very little financial support.

## Implementing solutions

Having decided what to do and what tactics to employ, the next question is 'how to implement these decisions?' Here the available literature is of one voice: *'Don't do it alone'*. Both Georgiades and Phillimore (1975) and Fairweather et al. (1974) emphasize very strongly the importance of creating a small group of approximately likeminded people who are all interested in seeing the organization change in a specific direction. This group should meet regularly and maintain close personal contact to offer one another mutual support. The cohesiveness and viability of this group determines, in large measure, the success of the change operation.

It is not particularly important who is in this group in terms of their formal status or power. Georgiades and Phillimore (1975: 317) suggest that often the best supporters of innovation and change are among the ranks of the people just below the top, where the personal commitment to the present is less, and where the drive for achievement may be higher, than at the very top. Top management should always be approached for their support, but a tacit agreement not to obstruct change is probably the best that can usually be hoped for. Fairweather et al. (1974: 108) similarly criticize the assumption that change is only possible through controlling the formal power structure. They found that the status of the original contact made in the organization was unrelated to whether or not change occurred. It seemed more important that whoever was involved was committed to change – in some form or another – rather than whether they held formal positions of power. Sometimes it is not easy to know exactly where 'power' resides. For example, the staff of health services are one of the most important resources that one is likely to be interested in influencing. As indicated earlier, there are approximately fifteen times as many nursing staff in mental hospitals as there are doctors. Thus, in this respect the nursing officer is at least as powerful as the doctor. (For rather different reasons the works manager and the catering officer also exert considerable influence and neither should they be ignored.) Georgiades and Phillimore also suggest that it may be important to work with those individuals who have some degree of freedom and discretion to manage their own affairs. They note that it profits little to work out an agreed change with someone who turns out not to have the authority to implement it. The guiding principles for implementation therefore seem to be: (1) work to produce an adopting group; (2) work to ensure that this adopting group is maintained; and (3) involve people in it from as many levels and parts of the organization as possible.

How can this group actually effect change? Firstly, they will need to work within the existing channels rather than outside them. At the outset the change group will not be powerful enough to stand on its own and therefore its members should exert their influence through the channels that already exist and that they are involved in. This means learning some of the skills necessary to cope with working in committees. Watts and Bennett (1983), see Chapter 4, pp. 95–6, have reviewed the research literature pertaining to the effective leadership of small groups of this kind and perhaps the most important conclusion that emerges is the desirability of combining analytic, structuring skills with emphatic, socially supportive skills. The effective leader is the person who has both qualities. This may be something of a 'tall order', but within the change group it may be that some individuals are good at one of these aspects of leadership and some are good at others. A division of labour may therefore be possible. The professional politicians also provide a wealth of hints on how to cope with committees. For example, Richard Crossman's diaries (Crossman 1979) contain innumerable examples of the principle of 'lobbying', i.e. ensuring that the members of the committee have been approached beforehand and their views canvased on a particular issue before it actually appears. He certainly did not believe that it was wise to leave it to chance that it will be 'alright on the day'. Crossman also notes the importance of those who control the written material presented to committees, i.e. the Minutes and the working reports. In his case this was usually the civil servants and he repeatedly complains of how they were able to exert undue influence on the discussion (op. cit.: 93–5). Thus, if you can be bothered to be the person who writes things down, you can have considerable control over what is discussed and hence what the outcome will be.

Social psychologists have also given some attention to the problems of how to achieve changes in attitudes and behaviour in a clinical context. Brehm (1976) reviews this evidence in relation to three prominent theories of attitude change, namely Reactance Theory, Cognitive Dissonance and Attribution Theory. She concludes that if enduring changes in attitude and behaviour are to occur then certain principles should be followed. These include: (1) give initial support to the client in his/her 'counter-attitudinal position', do not attempt to attack it 'head-on' and if there are two sides to the argument acknowledge it; (2) give the client maximum freedom in *choosing* to think and act differently, enduring change is most likely to occur if the client accepts personal responsibility with minimal external justification or coercion; (3) stress that it isn't going to be easy; and (4) isolate the change from future implications or consequences, suggest that it may be viewed as a trial or 'experiment' and that it doesn't necessarily commit the person to a permanent change of behaviour. These guidelines were formulated with the clinical situation in mind, i.e. persuading a patient to give up their symptoms; however, they are probably equally applicable to the process of organizational change. As indicated earlier, all change is likely to meet with some resistance and this is often based on an irrational fear that the person (or system) will be exposed as inadequate in the new situation. Since this fear is seldom actually rational, the parallel with the clinical situation is close.

Thus, the validity of opposing arguments and the difficulties of change should be acknowledged and people should be asked to choose a particular course of action, possibly on a trial basis at first. This is all good 'psychology', as well as being good professional practice.

## Feedback and evaluation

Those desiring institutional change may often be convinced of their own 'rightness' (they probably wouldn't be likely to embark on such a perilous undertaking unless they were). However, if they are also not open to being corrected, to being shown how this or that plan simply will not work, or is actually undesirable, then they run the risk, not only of alienating others, but also of failing to learn and change themselves. Pragmatism, flexibility and compromise are therefore essential. It is always wise to be satisfied with 'half-a-loaf' and not hold out for the 'perfect solution'; it seldom appears. Also, always be alert for when it is time to abandon a particular objective. Captains make fine figures going down with the sinking ship, but it's the rats who live to fight another day. Formal methods of feedback and evaluation may sometimes be possible through controlled trials or epidemiological data (see Ch. 3) and innovations in research design such as the development of time-series analysis (Cook and Campbell 1979) have made 'natural experiments' more possible. However, most change agents will have to rely on informal feedback and evaluation by the reports of others. Perhaps this should sometimes be biased in favour of seeing progress when little is there; reinforcement is often hard to come by (hence the importance of a mutually supportive group). But, in addition there should also be some 'objective' feedback and aspiring change agents should always seek the opinion of at least one or two relatively 'independent' observers.

One final word, all of those who have actually been involved in organizational change, whether from a research or a practical standpoint, have always concluded that it is an untidy, erratic, unpredictable business. The theoretical models of change as a systematic, gradual progression simply do not seem to hold in the real world (cf. Fairweather et al. 1974: 185). Tolerance of ambiguity and considerable patience are therefore essential attributes for change agents. Change is also usually slow, and Georgiades and Phillimore (1975: 315) note how it may be necessary to reappraise radically the time scale on which you usually work. Three to five years seem necessary for fundamental organizational change whether it is in industry, hospitals or schools. However, hero-innovators can be comforted by one fact: if you, or someone like you, does not change the organization it is unlikely that it will change by itself. To quote Fairweather et al. (1974: 185–6) once more, 'There is no evidence from the diffusion follow-up study that any appreciable degree of spontaneous adoption of innovation occurs in the absence of external stimulation somewhere in the process. The experimental data from the implementation phase also indicate that the outside intervention must be active, personal and often'. So, it is up to you. In the final analysis success will depend upon hard work, perseverance and, of course, a large slice of good luck.

## Summary

Creating the conditions for organizational change in health services depends upon a number of factors. Firstly, the change agent (or agents) must define the problem by understanding how and why patients move through the system of services, what changes are desirable and what effects these might have. This definition of the problem needs to be conveyed to the other people involved in delivering the service so that some kind of shared consensus as to what needs to be done is achieved. Next, initial goals should be set which are clear, specific and attainable. Subsequent progress and development can be evaluated with regard to an overall objective which is also clear, but may be less limited. The involvement of as many staff as possible in the change process is crucial at this stage, as in the Implementation phase. Implementation depends upon the creation of a viable and mutually supportive change group which needs to work initially through existing channels, persuading others by a mixture of political and psychological skills. The outcome of changes should be continuously monitored by informal means and by whatever formal methods are available. A willingness to learn from one's mistakes is essential. Flexibility, compromise and perseverance are also important attributes.

# Chapter 6

# Future directions

Up to now we have examined the care and rehabilitation of long-term psychiatric patients from an historical standpoint and through a consideration of what services are currently beginning to be made available for them and how these might best be organized and run. In this final chapter we will look towards the future and try to draw out some of the implications for research and practice of new ideas and changing social conditions. The first topic we will examine is 'Work'. Work and other kinds of structured activities have always played an important part in rehabilitation, but what implications do the present high levels of general unemployment have for the psychiatrically disabled? Why is work so particularly important for them and how can they be protected in the current climate? The importance of work is well established, but the importance of 'Coping', 'Social Networks' and 'Support' have only fairly recently begun to be appreciated. What are the implications of these new ideas in the context of psychiatric rehabilitation? How can they help us in the assessment, treatment and management of those with long-term disabilities? Finally, there is the issue of 'Prevention'. Community care is often justified by an appeal to its preventive possibilities, but how justified is such an appeal? How, and in what sense, can we expect that different patterns of service will actually *prevent* psychological and psychiatric disability? These are the questions to be considered here.

## Work

As indicated, the place of work in the history of psychiatric rehabilitation has been an important one. In Chapter 2 we saw how the reformers of the early nineteenth century came to believe that, 'a state of entire indolence and mental inertness is decidedly prejudicial to the patient' (p. 32). More recently the pioneering social psychiatrists of the post-war generation used work and other structured activities as one of the major means through which they transformed mental hospitals and began to offer chronic patients more normal and valued social roles (Bennett 1970; Clark 1974; Wing et al. 1964). At the present time we find ourselves faced with a situation of mass, and apparently structural, unemployment. The availability of the work role is becoming limited, even for the able-bodied, and if this situation is going to continue after the much hoped-for upturn in the economy occurs, then how will those with long-term psychiatric disabilities be affected? In the first place it is clear that they are likely to suffer the experience of unemployment earlier, and for longer periods, than their non-disabled counterparts. The employability of psychiatric patients has always been marginal and as the pool of available non-handicapped labour increases, so the disabled are squeezed further and further away from the boundaries of open employment. To understand what this means for the psychiatric patient, we need to understand the psychological – as well as the material – functions that work serves.

Bennett (1970), after Jacques (1967), has defined work as, 'the exercise of judgement or discretion within prescribed limits in order to reach a goal or objective' (op. cit.: 255). In this sense, he argues that work is different from traditional occupational or 'creative' therapies. In work the 'prescribed limits' are generally external, they represent the expectations of the employer, the consumer, or the 'market-place'. By contrast, in craft or creative therapies the demands are very much more internal, they consist of subjective judgements as to the worth of the final product. Thus, crafts may be useful in developing personal or aesthetic abilities, but they are less relevant to developing confidence in meeting expectations imposed from outside. Bennett suggests that one of the major therapeutic ingredients of work lies in this ability to present the individual with external challenges which, if they can be successfully mastered, provide a growth in confidence and self-esteem that can only effectively come from meeting the expectations of others.

Of course, this is not the only important difference between work and many of the other occupational or creative therapies often found in psychiatric hospitals. Work, as we have seen, imports a 'normal' role relationship into an abnormal setting. It can thus be an antidote to the prevailing culture of the hospital with its implicit emphasis on the 'sick-role'. Indeed, this was why it was introduced originally. Work can therefore have a 'normalizing' influence by offering patients an opportunity to function in something other than the sick-role. All 'therapies' have the danger of perpetuating sick-role relationships, since by definition 'therapy' is something that requires both a therapist and a patient. Thus, although therapy certainly has an important place in rehabilitation (see Ch. 1, p. 19) chronic patients are chronic *because* they have not responded well to attempts at treatment in the past. An overemphasis on 'therapeutic' activities may thus effectively prevent them from achieving more normal and independent social functioning.

An indication of how ability to work is used as an index of normality is noted by Wansbrough and Cooper (1980: 2–4). Thus, the question, 'Am I ready for work'? is still the crucial one in many patients' – and many professionals' – minds. It not only provides a passport out of hospital, but it is also an end in itself, a way of evaluating oneself socially and of defining oneself as 'normal' and therefore no longer 'ill'. If, as predicted, we are going to see a decline of work as a normal social activity over the next twenty years, then it will have to be replaced by some other criterion which is equally simple, equally clear cut, and had the same broad social appeal. At this time it is difficult to see what such a criterion might be. Without it the unemployed are almost certainly going to experience considerable difficulty in finding a role which offers them an acceptable status and social identity.

Thus far we have considered work as essentially an instrumental activity, i.e. a task that is completed in order to produce some product or goods, but this ignores its social component. Work is a *social* activity and it provides one of the most important sources of our social contacts and support. The importance of social functioning at work has been illustrated in a study by Watts (1978) who examined the outcome of a group of ex-psychiatric patients attending a vocational resettlement workshop. He found that those clients who eventually succeeded in securing and maintaining employment were rated during the training phase as socially more capable than their counterparts although they were indistinguishable in terms of their task (i.e. instrumental skill) performance. Thus, it was their social skills which seemed the critical determinant of their success. (This led me to become interested in methods of improving the social abilities of patients at work, see Shepherd 1977, 1978; Shepherd and Richardson 1979b.) Industrial tasks may also foster more co-operation, less dependence and greater social interaction, than traditional occupational therapies (Miles 1971, 1972).

One factor that work does have in common with more traditional methods of occupational therapy is the simple one of occupation, i.e. it provides a way of structuring and organizing time. This is important in relation to chronic psychiatric patients as they often have great difficulty in structuring and organizing time for themselves. It is not surprising that if one's internal world is disorganized and chaotic, then one is likely to experience difficulties in creating an external structure which gives order and a degree of predictability to daily life. The deleterious effects of failing to provide a clear structure and simple activities are well illustrated in the classic of Wing and Brown (1970). They found that the single most important factor discriminating between the three hospitals they studied was the time the patients spent doing nothing. This factor apparently directly influenced the levels of primary symptomatology observed. A similar conclusion has emerged regarding studies of schizophrenics in the community (see Ch. 3, pp. 51–2) where it has been shown that if face-to-face contact with over-emotional relatives could be reduced, and structured daytime activities provided, then the risk of symptomatic relapse is also greatly reduced. Simple structured activities, of which work is the best example, therefore provide a way of occupying and distracting patients and thus actually 'treating' their primary symptomatology. In the face of a poor response to drugs and other treatments, it may often be the only mechanism through which this can be achieved.

Of course, it is clear from the history of psychiatry that there are dangers in overemphasizing the importance of routine and regularity (cf. pp. 34–7). Social, recreational and leisure activities are also important, but it is difficult to ensure that they provide the kind of sustained activity that is necessary. There are simply few things that it is possible to engage in seven and half hours a day, five days a week! It must also be recognized that many patients may have very restricted social and leisure interests. For example, their major leisure activity may be watching television. (In this they are not abnormal as national surveys have shown that the average viewer watches at least 3–3½ hours per day, or in excess of 25 hours per week.) It may therefore be difficult to foster new leisure activities in individuals who lack both the interest and the motivation. It is also somewhat ethically dubious to attempt to foist on to mainly working-class patients the leisure and recreational interests of the educated middle-classes.

All these functions of work are 'latent', i.e. they are concealed within social structure of work, but of course work also has a manifest function – to earn money in order to purchase goods and services. Hartley (1980) has suggested that in this way 'work' and 'employment' may be distinguished. She suggests that the term 'work' may be used to refer to any activity which is purposeful, requires effort and discretion, has social significance and structures and organizes time, but does not necessarily involve a financial remuneration based upon the market value of the labour involved (e.g. education, child care, voluntary work). 'Employment' on the other hand may be used to refer to an economic exchange relationship between the employer and employee which usually takes place within the context of a larger organizational structure (an economy) and where the rewards are determined by the market value of labour. This is useful distinction as it allows us to argue that although we may not necessarily be able to provide *employment* for the psychiatrically disabled in the future, at least we may be able to offer them *work* and work substitutes (e.g. sheltered work, see below). 'Work', even without the strict economic contingencies of labour and reward, will still fulfil many of their basic psychological and social needs.

Of course, the need for basic economic support will still remain and the amount of this financial support, and the relationship between labour and reward within the context of a subsidized benefit system, are complicated and controversial issues. As we have seen, long-term psychiatric disability has always been closely associated with poverty and this is not surprising since, by definition, a long-term disability seriously impairs one's earning capacity. The disabled (psychiatric or otherwise) are therefore dependent upon external subsidies to maintain their living standards and this principle has been formally recognized ever since the seventeenth century. We may hope that in the future society will continue to support those who cannot support themselves at as high a level as possible. Once basic needs are met, the relationship between effort and reward is then a separate question. Obviously, there are dangers in erring on either side. If effort is great and reward is small then the individual is being exploited. Conversely, if effort is small but the rewards are proportionately large then there are dangers of reducing motivation, patronization, etc. There must be a balance between effort and reward, but where this balance should be struck is debateable. In sheltered work, or other work substitutes, a basic level of subsistence may be given 'non-contingently', with additional payments which are in some way more directly related to effort expended, e.g. incentive payments. It is a difficult balance to get right.

To summarize, work and work-like activities fulfil a number of important functions. They provide:

1 A sense of personal achievement and mastery through successfully mastering external challenges and meeting the expectations of others.
2 An opportunity to engage in 'normal', non-patient social roles and thus provide an antidote to the chronic sick-role.
3 An easily identifiable criterion of recovery from illness.
4 A sense of social status and identity.
5 Social contacts and support.
6 A means of structuring and occupying one's time.
7 Financial reward.

No other single activity is so rich and complex in its psychological, social and material significance. What does it mean therefore to be deprived of it? It is now widely recognized that unemployment constitutes a considerable stress for anyone and, for those with additional long-term psychiatric problems, these effects are more severe, more pervasive and more long-standing. The effects of unemployment in the general population have been well documented in a series of studies beginning with the classic work of Eisenberg and Lazarsfeld (1938) and continuing up to the present (see Jahoda 1979). Although there is now some controversy concerning the classic 'stage-theory' of unemployment, i.e. that all individuals pass through the same stages at the same rate, nevertheless there does seem to be general agreement on a characteristic progression. Firstly, the initial shock of unemployment is usually mitigated by a sense of relief that the crisis which has been impending for so long is now actually resolved. The newly unemployed may also be cushioned from the financial hardships of not working by redundancy payments, earnings-related benefits, etc. Thus, they are relatively free to pursue their search for a new job, or to engage in the leisure and recreational interests that full-time work has prevented them from doing. This 'honeymoon period', a kind of extended holiday, may make the newly unemployed wonder what all the fuss has been about. However, the holiday soon ends. Usually within about six months or so he/she is beginning to miss the structure and organization that work brought to their lives. If they cannot find another job quickly, and they cannot generate an alternative structure for themselves, they may begin to become disoriented and the normal rhythms of their life may become increasingly disrupted, e.g. their waking and sleeping patterns. They are also likely to become increasingly socially isolated since, as we have indicated, work is a very important source of friendships and without it social networks soon begin to contract. The unemployed person is also likely to experience some difficulty in locating themselves socially since the role of the unemployed is still somewhat ambiguous and he/she will need to redefine their social status and their relationship to others. Finally, as the financial pressure begin to bite so they cannot afford to maintain the leisure and interests they were able to previously, and their social withdrawal and inactivity become further compounded.

The short-term psychological effects of this disruption, alienation and withdrawal are well known. Depression, anxiety, anger, loss of self-esteem and feelings of helplessness are all common and at this stage the individual is likely to consult a GP and perhaps receive a prescription for minor tranquillizers. There are effects on the families too. Stokes (1982) found that within six months many of the unemployed men in his sample were showing a degree of anger, hostility and overassertiveness at home. He speculates that this may reflect an attempt to compensate for their losss of status and authority outside. As the situation becomes more chronic, so the alienation, social withdrawal and symptoms of psychological distress may become progressively more severe until after one year the individual joins the ranks of the long-term unemployed. At this point their chances of regaining employment are small.

It is worth noting in passing here that there are strong parallels between these social and psychological reactions to unemployment in those who have it forced upon them by economic changes and those who have it forced upon them by age (i.e. the retired) or by the demands of childcare (i.e. housewives). For example, the research of Brown and Harris (1978) mentioned earlier suggests that lack of work outside the home is one of the important factors leading to a higher risk of depressive symptoms in women. Thus, it may be argued with some justification, that the present preoccupation with the impact of general unemployment only serves to focus attention upon what has been the accepted situation for other disadvantaged groups for many years.

To return to the long-term unemployed, they are a large and seemingly intractable problem. At any one time they account for approximately one third of the total registered, i.e. currently more than a million, and despite some efforts to reduce their numbers they show little sign of decreasing. The reasons for this are not difficult to understand. Once unemployed for a substantial period of time the individual soon loses work 'habits' and may then find it difficult to readjust to the simple daily routine of work. The unemployed also no longer have any current references and this makes them an uncertain prospect for a prospective employer. They may have become somewhat withdrawn and socially anxious and are likely to be lacking in confidence. (Their social withdrawal also means that they become estranged from the most useful single source of finding work – word-of-mouth contact.) In addition they may have few skills, or skills that are no longer required. If, on top of all this, they also have the stigma of mental illness, their prospects are very bleak indeed. So what provisions exist to help them?

Vocational facilities for the psychiatrically disabled have been reviewed by Wansbrough (1981), Wansbrough and Cooper (1980) and Shepherd (1981b). Essentially they can be grouped under three main headings: (1) Hospitals, (2) Local Authority and Voluntary, and (3) the Manpower Services Commission (formerly the Department of Employment). Most large mental hospitals now have an Industrial Therapy Unit although, as we saw in Chapter 1, many of the old and new long-stay patients still remain unoccupied. Work in hospital is often dull and poorly paid, with seemingly little status attached to it. The dangers of exploitation are also considerable. What is needed is therefore a range of work activities, with some simple, repetitive tasks but some where more complex skills are also demanded (Bennett 1976b). In these days of increased growth in the service sector of the economy, clerical tasks might play an increasingly important part. It may also be possible to use some of the newer technologies to enable relatively unskilled workers to produce more sophisticated products, e.g. injection-moulding, silk-screen printing, etc. As Wansbrough (1981) notes, all patients should be given a chance to benefit from the experience of work, no matter how 'chronic' or apparently incompetent they might seem to be. But the most important battle still concerns the attitudes of staff. Doctors and nurses tend to believe that the sick need rest not labour and, in line with the 'therapy-orientation', staff are often much more interested in patients' emotional difficulties than their practical abilities to work and look after themselves.

Even in the 'community' similar attitudes may prevail. We saw in Chapter 3 how the majority of day services are still provided by the Health Authorities and how, within day care, very little provision is made for work activities (Edwards and Carter 1979: 46–7). Although there are some examples of good Local Authority provisions (Wansbrough and Cooper 1980: 41–6) for financial reasons, if for no other, it seems unlikely that local authorities are going to be able to make a very substantial contribution in the future. We may therefore have to look increasingly towards non-statutory provisions to meet these needs. The voluntary sector has made a very significant contribution to rehabilitation in the past by supplementing residential provisions with hostels, group homes, etc., perhaps in the future it will concentrate its efforts on supplementing day services, particularly with work-oriented provisions. There are already a number of examples of such ventures in existence, e.g. the Camberwell Rehabilitation Association, *Restore* in Oxford, and MIND's 'Portugal Prints' in London. It may be that one of the 'benefits' of the current recession is that more skilled engineers, managers, designers, etc. will be available with time and energy to devote to such projects. The statutory services might then be able to help with providing a proportion of staffing costs, rentals and other financial supports.

Money may also come from the Manpower Services Commission (MSC) although they have tended, quite understandably, to be preoccupied with other categories of long-term unemployed, notably the young and those who are more easily retrainable than long-term psychiatric patients. The MSC provisions for the psychiatrically disabled have always been limited by these other priorities. Thus, most Employment Rehabilitation Centres

(ERCs) operate a quota system restricting the number of places offered to psychiatric patients to 20–25 per cent. Similarly, the average length of stay at ERCs (8–12 weeks) is geared towards those who can adapt fairly quickly to new working environments and need only a brief period of reintroduction to work routines, or are looking for retraining in some new skill. Psychiatric patients, especially those with long-term difficulties, do not usually fall into either of these categories. However, the MSC has recently tried to respond to their special needs and there are now two ERCs which run longer training schemes (up to twelve months) specifically designed for the psychiatrically disabled. They are also funding a number of special projects in rehabilitation, but if Wing and Morris's (1981) national estimate of numbers of long-term patients is at all accurate (200,000) then the need for considerable additional provision is clear.

What the ERCs cannot provide, and perhaps what is most needed by psychiatric patients, is long-term sheltered work. The Remploy factories were set up to provide sheltered employment for all those with registered disabilities but again, for understandable reasons, the numbers of psychiatric patients have been restricted. Of the 8,000 or so total places, only approximately 2,000 are occupied by those with psychiatric disabilities (Wansbrough and Cooper 1980). These authors also note that of 87 factories surveyed in 1973, 25 per cent employed no mentally ill persons at all. The psychiatrically disabled are often difficult to supervise and less productive than other disabled groups and hence they may be unattractive to Remploy managers. But perhaps the major reason for their low numbers stems from their reluctance to join the disabled register. Nearly all large industrial concerns (including the Health Authorities) fail to employ their quota of 3 per cent disabled persons and this is undoubtedly partly due to the reluctance of those eligible to register. Psychiatric disability is perhaps a particularly unattractive label to attach to oneself voluntarily.

All this makes the job of the Disablement Resettlement

Officer (DRO) who is attached to each Job Centre especially difficult. While a patient does not necessarily need
to register to obtain the help of the DRO, if he/she does
not do so they must then accept competition on the open
market. It seems like 'heads-I-win-tails-you-lose': either
accept the stigma of registration, or face the stringencies
of open competition. The DRO is himself faced with pressures to place increasing numbers of unemployed in
decreasing numbers of places and cannot therefore be
blamed for concentrating on those with the best work
records and prospects. Perhaps a new kind of DRO,
specifically for the mentally ill, is required and there are
some precedents for such a post (see Wansbrough 1981:
88). The fundamental problem with the MSC's provisions
in relation to psychiatric rehabilitation is thus that, for
possibly understandable reasons, they have been primarily
*employment*-oriented rather than *work*-oriented. They
have been concerned with training, or retraining, suitable
candidates and returning them to the world of open
employment. As this world shrinks, especially as far as the
disabled are concerned, so this seems an increasingly
difficult and perhaps unrealistic aim. The psychiatrically
disabled need a range of work settings both in both
hospitals and in the community which can provide assessment, treatment and long-term management of their
disabilities at a number of different levels. This needs to
be done in specialized centres and with a much greater
number of places than is currently the case. As indicated
one of the great barriers to establishing these provisions
lies in the attitudes of the statutory services. Health
Authorities see themselves as in the business of providing
health services, not 'work services'. Similarly, Local
Authorities see themselves as providing social care and
support, but not necessarily employment. Finally, the
MSC is interested in work, but primarily in the form of
paid, open employment. As a consequence, none of the
statutory bodies may provide what is actually needed and
it may be left to the voluntary sector to offer work both

as a means of preserving health *and* as a social service.

One final point, we have stressed the need for a range of work activities in both hospitals and in the community. This is needed because of the wide range of abilities and backgrounds of our clients. Work need not be boring. But to make it interesting requires the participation of skilled people from outside the usual mental health professions. As indicated earlier, in these times of high unemployment one positive feature may be the availability of managers, excutives, designers, engineers, etc. who might be interested in using some of their skills in helping disabled people. They are a valuable resource and their possible contribution should not be overlooked. With such inputs there is also a much better chance that sheltered workshops and alternative ways of organizing work (e.g. co-operatives, etc.) may be made into viable and economically successful projects. If work is going to become a scarce commodity in the future, perhaps we might thereby try to ensure that those who need it most are deprived of it last, rather than first. Let us now turn our attention to some rather newer ideas and some very different problems.

## Coping, social networks and support

In contrast to the problem of work and unemployment, the ideas of coping, social networks and support have a relatively recent history in rehabilitation. They are also rather more theoretical concepts, but as we shall see they have some important practical implications. Of course, the concept of 'coping' is a familiar one from our everyday language, however it is only fairly recently that social scientists have begun to explore it in a more formal, technical sense. As specific techniques of behavioural treatment have developed so psychologists have also become increasingly interested in more general methods of coping with stressful and difficult situations. Hence, the concepts of self-control (Kanfer 1979) and the need to develop a repertoire of 'coping strategies' such as self-instruction, cue-controlled relaxation, self-generated goal-setting, anticipatory rehearsal, etc. (see Meichenbaum 1977). However, perhaps the most intensive study of coping strategies in the general population has been reported by Pearlin and Schooler (1978).

These authors define 'coping' as 'any response to external life strains that serves to prevent, avoid, or control emotional distress' (op. cit.: 3). On the basis of preliminary research they categorized potential 'life strains' (stressors) under four main headings: (1) *Marriage*; (2) *Parenting*; (3) *Household Economics*; and (4) *Occupation*. Examples of possible strains under each heading were:

1. Marriage – non-acceptance by spouse, non-reciprocity in the relationship, frustration of expectations;
2. Parenting – deviation of child's behaviour from parental standards, non-conformity of child to parents' values, disregard by child of parental status;
3. Household Economics – shortage of money, difficulty in meeting bills;
4. Occupation – inadequacy of rewards in work, noxiousness of work environment, overwork.

The effect of each specific area of stress was examined by asking subjects to indicate how much emotional distress it caused them. Thus, the interviewer might ask. 'Now adding up the good and bad points about your (job/marriage/etc.) how (bothered/tense/worried/etc.) do you feel?' The adjectives referring to emotional distress were selected on the basis of previous research as being particularly relevant to each area of stress and each was rated on a four point scale.

Coping responses were divided into three categories: 'Social resources' 'Psychological Resources' and 'Specific Coping Responses'. The first two categories referred to resources that were available to the person, rather than things that they actually did in order to cope. Hence, 'Social Resources' referred to the available network of social supports and contacts. 'Psychological Resources' to the inner resources of an individual's personality and 'Specific Coping Responses' to the various cognitive and behavioural techniques that they actually used to cope with stressors. In this paper Pearlin and Schooler concentrated on Psychological Resources and Specific Coping Responses and did not consider Social Resources (see pp. 137–40 below). Under the heading of 'Psychological Resources' they include such personality factors as positive self-esteem, negative self-denigration and the degree of a sense of personal mastery. They measured these factors using simple self-report questionnaires. Under the heading of 'Specific Coping Responses' they found seventeen factors covering the four different areas of potential stress which could be grouped under three main headings: (1) responses which attempted to *change* the situation, e.g. negotiation in marriage, punitive discipline in parenting, active job-seeking in occupation; (2) responses which attempted to *re-evaluate* the stress, e.g. making positive comparisons ('count your blessings') or selective abstraction ('look on the bright side'); and (3) responses which attempted simply to *manage* the stress, e.g. 'everything will work out for the best in the end', 'what can't be

*Fig. 1* Relationship between life strains, coping and stress

| Life strains (stressors) × | Coping mechanisms = | Stress (emotional distress) |
|---|---|---|
| e.g. – Marital<br>– Parental<br>– Household Economics<br>– Occupational | e.g. – Social Resources<br>– (social networks, support, etc.)<br>– Psychological Resources (self-esteem, mastery, self-denigration)<br>– Specific Coping Responses (change, re-evaluation, management) | e.g. – Unhappiness<br>– Worry<br>– Tension<br>– Frustration |

cured must be endured', etc. Again, the Specific Coping Responses which comprised each factor were assessed using simple self-report questionnaires. So, we have a model for analysing the coping process which is summarized in Figure 1 above.

Life strains operate on the individual to produce emotional distress, but the effect of stressors is mediated by the influence and availability of various coping mechanisms. Pearlin and Schooler examined how these coping mechanisms affected this stress-distress relationship in a community sample of 2,300 people living in urban Chicago. They analysed the results using a complex multivariate statistical procedure (stepwise regression) and this enabled them to identify how each coping mechanism effectively blocked the relationship between specific stressors and self-reported distress.

The results of this elaborate and fascinating study are complicated, but a number of important conclusions emerged, viz:

1. *Do Specific Coping Responses succeed in reducing the effects of stress?* The answer to this question is 'it depends'. Specific Coping Responses do succeed in reduce the effects of stress in some areas (Marriage and Parenting) but not in others (Household Economics and Occupation). The authors explain this finding by suggesting that in areas such as Household Economics and Occupation the stresses are shaped by largely impersonal forces outside the individual's own direct control. Hence, active attempts to cope with stress by trying to change the situation are unlikely to be effective. Conversely, in areas such as Marriage or Parenting stress depends on much more interpersonal factors which may be more directly influenced and changed.

2. *Which Specific Coping Response is most effective?* In general, the difference between specific coping responses is small. However, in those areas where they do make an appreciable difference (Marriage and

Parenting) a degree of self-reliance, as opposed to a reliance on others, surprisingly emerges as being consistently important. Also, a positive attempt to seek a solution to problems in interpersonal relationships or regarding children seem more effective than simple confrontation or ventilation of feelings. In areas where the effects of specific coping responses were less overall (Household Economics and Occupation) the most effective types of coping involved the manipulation of goals and values, i.e. the re-evaluation and management of stress. Thus, some impersonal unremitting stresses demand a capacity to endure rather than to change. In general, the more varied the individual's repertoire of coping responses the more likely they were to be effective in reducing distress. Thus, for example in marriage the effects of stress were virtually eliminated in people who reported using 5 or 6 different specific coping responses.

3. *Do Psychological Resources succeed in reducing the effects of stress*? Here again, it depends. As before the greatest amelioration of stress through psychological resources is seen in the areas of Marriage and Parenting. However, even in Household Economics and Occupation some positive benefits of having good psychological resources are to be seen.

4. *Which Psychological Resources are most important*? Here the picture is a little clearer than regarding specific coping resources. An absence of self-denigration, i.e. not having a negative attitude towards oneself, consistently emerges as the most useful psychological resource to possess. A sense of positive 'mastery', i.e. a feeling that one has some control over the forces shaping one's life, is the second most important. Positive self-esteem, i.e. a definitely favourable attitude towards oneself, is the least important.

5. *Which is most important, Specific Coping Responses or Psychological Resources*? What people do, or what people are? Again, the answer depends on what kind

of stress is considered. In Marriage specific coping responses are much more important than psychological resources; in Parenting they are equally important; in Household Economics psychological resources are more important than coping responses; and in the area of Occupation neither makes much difference. Thus, different kinds of coping mechanisms seem to be effective against different kinds of stress.

6. *Are any other variables important*? Pearlin and Schooler also examined whether any background demographic variables in their sample (age, sex, social class) were associated with the use of more positive coping mechanisms. Interestingly, they found that while age was not related, sex and social class were. Thus, women and those who were poorer and less educated tended to possess fewer postitive coping mechanisms. They note from this that not only are certain sections of our society disadvantaged in social and economic terms, they may also be socialized in ways that equip them less adequately to deal with the stresses and strains they are likely to encounter.

This is a highly original study and is of considerable interest and importance. It represents one of the few attempts to understand how ordinary people cope with the stresses of everyday life and it has some exciting and novel implications for the practice of rehabilitation. The authors acknowledge that the research has a number of limitations. For example, we do not know whether their conclusions can be generalized to other samples in other situations. Would a similar picture emerge if we studied specifically schizophrenics, or those with long-term depressive disorders? We cannot be sure, but there is now evidence to suggest that at least some of their findings may also apply to other clinical groups. Thus, Litman et al. (1979) found that the possession of a variety of coping styles discriminated most effectively between alcoholics who did or did not relapse into drinking. Results by Litman et al. also seemed to confirm the importance of positive and reflective thinking as an effective coping response. However, the effectiveness of different kinds of coping mechanisms for different clinical groups requires further investigation. Pearlin and Schooler's study also examined only a relatively restricted range of stressors and we might ask whether other situations are more stressful, or stressful in different ways, for different groups? Finally, as they indicate, they have only investigated a small number of potential specific coping responses and psychological resources. With a little ingenuity one can think of a whole range of possible alternative responses and psychological resources relevant to particular client groups, e.g. social withdrawal as a coping response in schizophrenia; engagement in pleasurable activities as a coping response in depression, etc.

Perhaps what this study offers us above all is a conceptual model for investigating 'coping' and some clues as to the effectiveness of specific coping mechanisms for specific stresses. Hopefully, other researchers will build upon Pearlin and Schooler's work and begin to identify the specific kinds of coping mechanisms which are effective in reducing distress caused by particular stressors in particular populations. We might even speculate that a time will come when routine assessments for rehabilitation will include a consideration of the individual's available coping mechanisms, their range and flexibility, and the kinds of stresses he/she has to encounter. This might lead to therapeutic interventions aimed at fostering specific coping responses (as in Kanfer 1979; Meichenbaum 1977) or simply a concentration on developing a variety of coping mechanisms. The evidence seems quite compelling that possessing a number of coping responses is preferable to relying on one or two and this gives us a very different perspective to the traditional 'single treatment' model. Coping is obviously a complex, multidimensional construct and as yet we have only begun to scratch its surface. As Pearlin and Schooler note, they did not consider Social Resources (networks and support) and so let us now go on to examine these in more detail.

The idea that a person's network of social contacts provides psychological support and helps them cope with adversity is again a 'common-sense' notion. However, it has received surprisingly little attention from mental health professionals. They have often been more concerned with intra- and inter- personal dynamics and it is only fairly recently that 'social support' has been the subject of serious research. An important paper which marked the resurgence of interest in this area was by Henderson (1977) entitled *The Social Network, Support and Neurosis: The Function of Attachment in Adult Life*. In this paper Henderson argued that social networks provide the means whereby we obtain that complex commodity commonly, but unsatisfactorily referred to, as 'support'. He suggested that, particularly in times of stress, the availability of emotionally positive interactions with others provides a degree of protection against psychological, perhaps even physical, disorders. His research team then went on to develop a structured interview method (The Inverview Schedule for Social Interaction – ISSI) based on a theoretical paper on the nature of social relationships by Weiss (1974). (For a full description of the ISSI, its rationale and scoring, see Henderson 1980; Henderson et al. 1980a; Duncan-Jones 1981). The ISSI is designed to provide a systematic examination of an individual's primary group, i.e. that network of social contacts with whom he/she has both regular face-to-face contact and some apparent degree of commitment. This entails listing, in rank order, all those persons with whom the subject reports an emotionally close relationship ('Attachment figures') and examining in some detail the nature and adequacy of these relationships. A similar set of items covers the availability and adequacy of friends, work associates and other, more casual social contacts. Changes in the social network over time are assessed and also the presence of emotionally unpleasant attachments. The interview schedule is lengthy and complicated and it has been the subject of painstaking development by the research team. However, a number of studies have now been reported using it which demonstrate a clear inverse relationship between the presence of good social supports and various neurotic symptoms in both out-patient and community samples (Henderson et al. 1978b, 1980b). Similar results have been reported by Miller and Ingham (1976) and in Goldberg and Huxley (1980). Also, Brown and Harris's (1978) work (Ch. 3, p. 65) suggested an increased vulnerability to depressive symptoms in women who do have a confiding support available. Finally, Liem and Liem (1978) have argued that one of the most important factors influencing the relationship between social class and mental illness (apart from unemployment) is the presence or absence of social supports.

All these studies highlight the close connection between social supports and mental health problems. However, before we could use them as a basis for interventions aimed at improving levels of social support, we need to know (a) exactly what it is about 'support' that is supportive, and (b) whether there is a true causal connection between support and mental health, i.e. does lack of support actually 'cause' mental illness? Or, does mental illness lead to a failure to obtain supportive relationships? (Or, are both the product of some 'third variable'?)

With regard to the nature of social support we have already seen that it is necessary to make a distinction between the quantitative and qualitative aspects of social contact. Thus, it is not simply the *number* of available social relationships, but also their *quality* that is important. This point has been made particularly clearly by Heller (1979) where he discusses the paradox that close interpersonal ties can sometimes be positive and sometimes negative. In this connection, we saw earlier in Chapter 3 how schizophrenic and depressed patients may have very different social needs. In the former case, their needs are often met by simply providing 'company', somewhere where they can go and be with people without necessarily engaging in close relationships. (Indeed, schizophrenics may actually need to avoid over-involved or over-critical relationships.) Conversely, depressives have a much greater need for intimate and confiding relationships and perhaps a greater sensitivity to feeling lonely. It is interesting to speculate that these diagnostic differences may also reflect underlying sex differences. Thus, close confiding relationships seem generally more important for women (depressives) than for men (schizophrenics), see Horwitz (1977). So, before we can begin to use measures of social networks and support as part of our routine assessments for rehabilitation, we need to know exactly what kinds of social networks we should be focusing upon. The critical dimension which defines different networks, e.g. 'the network of people that I can talk to whenever I have a problem' or 'the network of places that I can go to and just be with people and feel comfortable', will be different for different individuals depending on the kinds of social support that they most need.

Thus, in the future we might hope to see rehabilitation workers not only concerned with assessing and developing patients' coping repertoires, but also their social networks and their needs in terms of support. This implies the development of much shorter and simpler methods than the research instruments currently available. A great deal more work also needs to be done in understanding the influence that these factors have on other aspects of outcome, e.g. admission to hospital, maintenance of relationships, the capacity to withstand life-events, etc. When this has been achieved we will then be able to evaluate the effectiveness of different intervention strategies aimed at enhancing coping skills, social networks, or the quality of support. All this constitutes an exciting set of prospects, but in the meantime for many professionals there remains the persistent feeling that perhaps this laborious process could be circumvented by some kind of more radical social and political change. Is this just a 'pipe-dream'? Or, are there some limited senses in which it can be made a reality?

## Prevention

Prevention is truly the 'glittering prize' of mental health. The move towards care in the community has often been used to argue that if a more radical restructuring of the 'community' were to take place, then perhaps the need for systems of care would be very much less, if not even completely abolished. How realistic are such claims? How, and in what sense, can 'community care' be preventative? After Caplan (1964) we must first distinguish between three different types of prevention: Primary, Secondary and Tertiary. Primary prevention is what most people would see as 'true' prevention, i.e. a reduction in the incidence of new cases of a particular condition occurring in a given population at a given point in time. This is the 'public-health' model. In order to achieve effective primary prevention we require two conditions: (1) an accurate knowledge of the cause (or causes) of disease states, and (2) the means to eradicate these causes at source. The classic example of primary prevention is the advance in public health achieved through an understanding of the relationship between diseases and infections of the water supply and hence the consequent improvements in plumbing and sanitation. Other examples would be vaccination programmes, control of the malarial mosquito, etc. How feasible is such an approach in the context of psychiatric rehabilitation?

In the first place, it is clear that we possess little in the way of accurate knowledge as to the initial causes of psychiatric disability. We can speculate about the influence of family and social factors, unemployment, poverty, and so on, but we have little direct evidence as to their *aetiological* significance. Conditions like schizophrenia and major affective disorders are complex states where a multiplicity of genetic, biochemical, psychological, social and environmental factors all play their part. To talk of simple causes, or even the same pattern of causes invariably leading to similar outcome, is clearly a nonsense.

At a broader social and political level a similar lack of evidence is apparent. Thus, if the broad cultural and political characteristics of a society made an appreciable difference to the incidence of major mental illnesses one might expect to find societies and political arrangements where such conditions did not occur, or at least were exceedingly rare. In fact, this does not seem to be the case. The World Health Organization's multinational study of schizophrenia indicates that a condition, clearly recognizable as schizophrenia, occurs all over the world from North America to Nigeria and from Soviet Russia to central India (Jablensky and Sartorius 1975; Sartorius et al. 1977). In an extensive review of social and cultural influences of psychopathology Dohrenwend and Dohrenwend (1974) conclude that there is little evidence to support the 'noble savage' hypothesis or the idea that 'a simple and relatively uncomplicated way of life provides virtual immunity from mental disorders' (op. cit.: 430). Of course, this does not mean that the actual content of symptomatology does not differ across cultures. The delusional content of a schizophrenic's ideas in Nigeria may be very different from his/her counterpart in Washington. Nevertheless, both are clearly suffering from schizophrenia. (Nor does it also imply that some cultures don't produce their own unique, and sometimes rather exotic, forms of psychopathology, e.g. *koro*, see Dunham 1976.) Dohrenwend and Dohrenwend's (1974: 433) review also produces evidence to suggest that there may not actually have been a substantial increase in the incidence of major psychiatric disorders over time. We saw in Chapter 2 how concerned the Victorians were about the stresses and strains of 'modern' society and the evidence from American hospital records of the 1840s indeed suggests that there may not have been a great increase in the actual incidence rates of functional psychoses over the past 100 years.

All this evidence therefore indicates that we have few grounds to embark upon a wholesale programme of social and political reconstruction which is justified on the basis of eradicating major mental illnesses. (Of course, this is not to say that social and political change may not be justified for other reasons.) One might also question the ethics of mental health professionals who engaged themselves in such a task. Such changes, even if justified by empirical evidence, would have ramifications far beyond the mental health arena and would thus take them well outside their spheres of competence and responsibility. This is not to say that mental health professionals should not be involved in social and political reform in so far as it affects them as ordinary citizens. But it is very different to be involved in political issues as a member of the 'body politic' as opposed to being involved as a member of some professional body. This distinction between personal and professional political responsibility is an important one and we should always strive to avoid giving spurious credibility to what are essentially personal statements by an appeal to professional affiliations. Having said all this, there are still some areas of social change where professional and political interests may coincide, but these are more often in the area of Secondary prevention.

Secondary prevention refers not to a decrease in the *incidence* of new cases in a population, but to a reduction in their *prevalence* through early identification and the application of more rapid and effective forms of treatment and management. Hence, many of the topics which have been central this book can be seen within this context. The whole concept of care in the community represents an attempt to intervene more effectively with those who are already identified as having potential long-term mental health problems and to provide them with more effective forms of treatment and management. To the extent that their disabilities can be minimized so their prevalence should be reduced. We saw in Chapter 3 that there is now considerable evidence that care in the community can be effective in this sense and that minimizing the use of hospital admission and providing alternatives on a community basis can help reduce many of the secondary, and some of the tertiary, handicaps of the psychiatrically disabled.

It is therefore interesting to note that the international studies of schizophrenia lend support to the idea that broad social and cultural factors do play an important part in influencing the course and outcome of established mental illnesses. Thus, Sartorius et al. (1977) present results concerning a two year follow-up of various groups of schizophrenic patients which show a considerably better outcome for those from centres in developing countries (e.g. India, Columbia, Nigeria) compared with those from centres in the so-called 'developed countries' (e.g. Sweden, United Kingdom, Russia and North America). It seems that although broad social and cultural factors may not make much of a difference to the incidence of major mental illnesses, they may make a difference to their course and outcome. Such findings have led Cooper and Sartorius (1977) to speculate that in modern industrialized societies schizophrenics face a whole range of disadvantages (stigmatization, lack of opportunities for employment, lack of family support, etc.) which are considerably less in undeveloped countries. They relate these differences in social structures to increased industrialization, increased specialization in industry, and increased mobility leading to a disruption of extended family networks. Attempts to educate the public regarding mental health, providing sufficient suitable sheltered employment, securing adequate resources to support families who are caring for the long-term mentally ill, are therefore all objectives which have a strong political element and which may be fairly easily justified by an appeal to their *secondary* preventative effects.

One final point regarding secondary prevention. We saw in Chapter 1 how long the long-term mentally ill are a very specialized sub-group of the total population who suffer with psychological and psychiatric problems. They

are also often an unattractive group as far as the professionals are concerned because of their difficulty and their
lack of responsiveness to treatment. In addition, they have
little social or economic status or power. But they are
important because they make such extensive demands on
the services. All these factors lead to the danger that, in
the desire to economize on services, resources will be
diverted away from the hospital (beds closed, etc.) but
instead of being used to develop alternative services in
the community for those patients so deprived, these
resources will be spent on providing extra services to
groups who are already in the community and who are
more 'attractive', i.e. less 'chronic' more treatable and
more co-operative. Such developments may then be
justified by an appeal to their 'preventive' value with
regard to some kind of global concept of 'mental illness'
while in reality they offer nothing to the long-term
mentally ill except a further diminution of services.

To guard against this danger we must continually
remind ourselves that the psychiatric morbidity at a
primary health care level consists mainly of minor affective disorders and chronic neuroses (see Ch. 1 pp. 2–4)
and that these conditions are rarely, if ever, admitted to
hospital. Developing primary health care services in the
community may be a desirable end in itself but it is
unlikely to serve any useful function, preventative or
otherwise, as far as the *long-term* mentally ill are
concerned. If one wants to develop preventative services
for them, one needs to remain in close contact with the
settings where they are to be found in the greatest concentrations, i.e. the acute admission wards of the mental
hospital, or the psychiatric ward of the District General
Hospital. The community-based services (day care,
hostels, domiciliary visiting, etc.) must therefore link to
these services and not, in the first instance, to primary
health care. All long-term patients may have a General
Practitioner, but only a small minority of those with
psychological problems who consult their GPs are long-

term. If rehabilitation in the community is to have a chance of succeeding in preventing long-term disabilities we must ensure that what little resources it does have are not used to improve the care of different client groups.

Tertiary prevention is the attempt to minimize the accumulation of chronic disabilities which accrue through poor treatment or inefficient management. We have already argued that a community-based rehabilitation service is likely to be superior to a hospital-based service in this respect, although we have also seen how the re-location of a service is no simple guarantee that its effectiveness will also be increased. Health services exist to promote health, and at the very least they may aim to treat people without actually doing them harm in the process. Many of our old-fashioned mental hospitals seemed almost designed to increase disability and as long as community-based services don't fall into the same trap, by neglect possibly rather than by design, perhaps the long-term mental patient may be able to look forward to a slightly rosier future.

## Summary and concluding comments

In this small book we have examined some very large problems. It is not easy to pick out the most important points, but nevertheless some conclusions do seem to stand out.

In the first place, the long-term mentally ill are a relatively small, but highly prominent, group. Compared with the rest of psychiatry they have a unique set of characteristics which makes them both difficult to 'treat' and yet a problem to 'manage'. They do not fit easily within traditional medical concepts like *disease* and *cure* and their problems appear much more like longstanding difficulties in social adaptation rather than mental 'illnesses'. They may not be curable in the usual sense of the word and yet treatment is still an integral part of their management.

The history of their care is a history of disadvantage.

Disadvantaged in social and economic terms, their ability to command a good quality of care has always been limited. Disadvantaged in personal and psychological terms, their ability to attract sustained professional interest and resources has always been erratic. They have therefore existed at the mercy of philanthropic patrons or governments. Care in the community, which is now fashionable, represents in many ways a return to pre-industrial practices. It is an enigmatic jigsaw whose pieces may, or may not, eventually fit together to the benefit of those that it is meant to serve. It will certainly not succeed if it is not given adequate resources to do so.

At the moment day services are at the centre of this puzzle, but a good quality of care will certainly not be bought simply by relocating the services. High quality care is a complex goal and it consists of a number of elements each of which is a necessary, but not sufficient, condition for its attainment. Standards of care also depend ultimately upon the qualities of the staff involved and supporting them is therefore one of the most important tasks. Services also need to be co-ordinated and the 'illusion of comprehensiveness' thereby maintained. This illusion is like a mirage in reverse, i.e. it is not an apparently tangible object which turns out to be illusory, but rather a vague and superficially flimsy network of services which turns out to be an efficient and co-ordinated whole. Whether this is achieved depends not only upon the resources that are provided (money, buildings, staff, etc.) but also upon a degree of vision and an optimism that change *is* possible. These in turn depend upon mutual support by interested professionals and the maintenance of an informed, and involved, consensus.

The future holds many possibilities. There is room for exciting new developments in the practice of psychiatric rehabilitation, but the challenges of changing patterns of general economic and social life must also be faced. Perhaps a fault of this book is that we have stressed repeatedly what 'might', and 'should' be, rather than 'what is'. However, without a clear understanding of what is possible, we will not progress beyond what we have now. Whether this progress will remain only in the realm of 'possibility', time alone will tell.

# A case example

There now follows a case example of rehabilitation. This case illustrates many of the important themes which have been touched upon in this book. It is a shortened version of a chapter by the author entitled 'Planning the rehabilitation of the individual' published in F. N. Watts and D. H. Bennett, *Theory and Practice in Psychiatric Rehabilitation*, published by John Wiley & Sons Ltd (1983). It appears with the kind permission of the editors and the publishers and this is gratefully acknowledged.

John is 24 years old, he has been referred to a Day Hospital for 'assessment and rehabilitation' at the initial request of his parents. The main problem seems to be that John has great difficulty in holding down a job for longer than about six months. His instability in work has been markedly worse in the last four years. Since leaving school, when aged 17, he has actually had seven jobs, the longest being as a clerk in the Post Office lasting 10 months. He has usually been sacked rather than leaving work voluntarily and his employers have complained of his slowness and repeated instances of 'childish' behaviour. At the initial interview he seems quite a pleasant young man, he looks a bit nervous and tends to smile rather a lot when asked about his problems. His parents are present at this interview and father seems rather quiet while mother does most of the talking. She seems very worried about John's failure at work and keeps asking what will be done to help him.

In some ways John's case is not a typical one. He does not fit the traditional stereotype of the psychiatric rehabilitee, thus he has not already spent long periods in hospital and he actually seems to show little in the way of recognizable psychiatric symptoms. But John is perhaps an example of a new kind of problem for psychiatric rehabilitation. His difficulties are not hidden under the effects of institutionalization and his problems seem to be due to social and environmental factors rather than to 'illness'. Irrespective of whether John is a chronic schizophrenic, or simply a rather inadequate young man, we must begin with a thorough assessment of his difficulties.

Assessments should be both valid and reliable. That is, they should measure adequately whatever it is that we are interested in, and they should do this in a reproducible way. At this stage a comprehensive coverage of the possible problems (content validity) is what is most important. When specific problems have been identified, more detailed and reliable measures can be taken. The first problem to consider is the patient's 'engagement' in the service. This is particularly important in community-based rehabilitation where poor attendance and high drop-out rates are relatively common. In John's case attendance was not a problem, but staff must always be alert to those who don't attend and be prepared to act. This need to respond quickly means that this is a task which cannot easily be left to one specialized professional group (e.g. Social Workers or Community Nurses) and all staff involved in rehabilitation must be prepared (and encouraged) to go into the community. This in turn implies having good contacts with the patients' families, and it will be noted that John's parents were invited to his initial interview. A relationship can then be built up between the staff and others who have some significance in the patient's life so that, at the very least, staff will have some idea of what might be happening to the patient when they are not attending. An understanding of this may lead to a negotiation over various aspects of his / her programme. For example, some kind of part-time arrangement may be necessary for some patients in the initial stages. Similarly, special working conditions (e.g. working alone), temporary exemption from an aspect of the programme (e.g. group), or special attention from certain staff members on arrival, may all help an anxious or withdrawn patient settle down and become attached. Other kinds of family interventions aimed at improving non-attendance will be discussed later.

The next questions concern physical and psychiatric symptoms. Physical status is always important to check, especially for those patients who have spent long periods in hospital. Basic physical functions like sight, hearing and condition of the teeth need to be looked at carefully if one is thinking about how he/she is going to manage at work or in the community. The provision of appropriate prosthetic devices such as spectacles, hearing aids, and dentures can often be just as crucial as the effective control of symptoms. A brief check of psychiatric symptoms should follow next and here the doctor in the team obviously has the central role to play. However, other members of staff may also be able to give the doctor information about how the patient appears in other contexts, e.g. at work and at home, and this may be very important in arriving an accurate diagnosis. Thus, a patient may appear withdrawn and apathetic in one setting but relatively lively and outgoing in another. We should always be cautious about assessing psychiatric symptoms, or any other problems, by interview alone and we should aim to incorporate as many observations as possible from other sources. In John's case very few symptoms could be elicited by interview; his problems were evident in other situations.

The next set of possible problems to consider concern the patient's attitude towards their illness (the secondary disabilities). For many patients the meaning they make of their illness experience can represent more of an obstacle to their rehabilitation than any primary symptoms, or indeed any loss of skills. Patients may wish to deny the reality of their difficulties and maintain fixed and unrealistic expectations. At the other extreme, they may come to see themselves as completely disabled and capable of nothing but a permanent, dependent, 'sick' role. Sometimes, the existence of these secondary disabilities can only be inferred from the patient's behaviour. For example, by repeated avoidance or non-compliance with treatment plans. On other occasions, as in the refusal to take medication, the wish to deny and avoid the reality of difficulties may be much clearer. Some patients may be so frightened of becoming 'ill' again that they wish to avoid all stress and therefore will not co-operate in any treatment programme. Although John had never suffered a psychiatric illness as such, he did not seem particularly interested to examine why he was having difficulties, or to look at ways in which he could change. His parents were genuinely perplexed. They kept asking if he should be labelled as 'ill' and what implications this would have for what could be expected of him. These problems of motivation and the attitudes of key relatives are crucial.

We come next to the problems associated with the skills necessary to survive as an independent person in the community. The adequacy and the stability of the patient's current accomodation need to be considered, as does his/her financial situation. Money is an obvious factor in motivation, especially as far as work is concerned, and yet it is easily overlooked. We also need information about basic educational skills and this is one of the few areas in which formal psychological tests may be useful. The patient needs to be assessed with regard to basic self-care skills, e.g. personal hygiene, care of clothes, and we need to know if they can cook for themselves, if they can look after their accommodation, if they can find their way about in the community and use public transport, shops the post office, etc. All these kinds of problems require assessment by direct observation and they should not be assessed by simple, uncorroborated interviews or self-report. Again, they depend on staff who are able to observe the patients directly in the community or in a realistic, simulated environment in hospital, e.g. 'home-management' areas

It is particularly important with these kinds of problems to separate out what are deficits in *skills* and what are deficits in *motivation*. For example, John was quite well able to look after himself, his educational skills were good and he had few problems in coping with all the basic aspects of self-care when he was asked to perform under supervision in the day hospital. However, when he and his parents were questioned it became clear that he actually did very little of this when at home. His parents managed nearly all his affairs for him including his money, even buying his clothes. His problems were therefore not due to a lack of skills, but a lack of motivation. This is a crucial distinction for, as we shall see later, it has important implications for the kinds of interventions that one might consider later.

The next area to consider is work. Here we need rating scales which cover all the relevant aspects of work behaviour (including the social factors) and we also need a realistic work setting and good observers such that the assessments can be made validly and reliably. It must be remembered that the accuracy of assessments is determined by the setting and the extent to which the observers share a common frame of reference as well as by the characteristics of the assessment instrument. Hence, if observers share a commonly mistaken idea of what they should be looking for, they can agree and therefore be reliable, but still be 'wrong' in the sense of not being valid. To provide a valid assessment of work performance we therefore not only require a realistic physical environment, we also require a realistic social environment in the sense of realistic expectations. Mental health professionals may find it difficult to provide these kinds of expectation, since they may lack the necessary experience. Thus, volunteers or professionals from industries settings may need to be recruited to improve the validity of the assessments that can be made.

John was set to work in the clerical office. When he was observed his problems began to become apparent. He quickly established himself as the office 'fool' and was slow and made inane comments. He was seldom observed to out instructions and created a general impression of slackness and unreliability. Although initially both staff and patients were vaguely amused by this behaviour, after a short time they became irritable and lost patience with him. When confronted with this, he admitted his mistakes but just grinned nervously. In his social interactions with both peers and supervisors he seemed timid and unassertive and seldom initiated any contact. He tended to ask unnecessary questions, repeat back what others had said and made insane comments. He was seldom observed to put forward an opinion or state a personal goal or aim for the future. In order to rule out the possibility that John's behaviour could be explained by intellectual deficits his intelligence was assessed and he was found to be functioning towards the top end of the average range. There was no evidence of any other cognitive problems. In order to assess his social difficulties in more detail he was asked to take part in role-play sessions with one or two of the staff. To everyone's surprise he demonstrated that he could produce appropriate social behaviour, including assertive responses, in these role-play sessions.

By now we were beginning to build up a picture of John's difficulties, of what they were and of where they occurred. We were beginning to see how they interfered with his functioning and we had some clues as to what interventions might be necessary. But, there is one important area that we had not yet considered. This was the nature of his family situation and his social supports outside the day setting. We decided to see John and his family at home and two members of staff (a doctor and a nurse) made a series of visits. Assessing family functioning is a difficult and controversial area. Theories abound and it is not at all clear which theory provides the most useful conceptual framework. However, a number of basic questions should be considered. First, there is the issue of roles and responsibilities, who does what? It may be important to know in some detail who does the various chores, who cooks the meals, puts out the rubbish, takes care of the children, etc. What are the domestic roles and does everybody have one? The next question, which follows on from the first, is how did this particular pattern of roles and responsibilities arise? In any family there are bound to be conflicts and disagreements and these often focus around who is responsible for which tasks. How are these conflicts and disagreements resolved? How much is there of 'positive' and 'negative' problem-solving? (Positive problem-solving consists of making constructive suggestions, offering alternatives, compromising, etc.; whereas negative responses include criticizing, complaining, denying responsibility). We move on next to consider the family structure in terms of power, 'alliances' and the recognition of individual autonomy. Who seems particularly close to whom? Is each person given some 'space' to themselves? Emotional expression is the next area and here one needs to look very carefully at the levels of anger, criticism, hostility as well as love, affection and sometimes overprotection which each member expresses for one another. In addition to the nature and amount of emotional expression, it is also important to consider its clarity. Some recent research has focused on possible discrepancies between the intended content of communications and their received impact. For example, it has been shown that in distressed couples communications are often received much more negatively than is intended. This suggest the influence of cognitive 'sets' or 'stereotypes', filtering the information prior to it being perceived. These stereotypes are the family 'myths', e.g. 'he's hopeless';

'she's the clever one' etc. They are built up over years and may be highly resistant to disconfirming evidence. This brings us to the final area, the family's attitude towards 'outsiders'. What are their attitudes to people outside the family and to professionals? Are they relatively welcoming and open, or rather suspicious and self-sufficient? The family's attitude towards how they deal with problems will be an important factor determining how easy they are to engage in some kind of family work.

John's family was an interesting one. We have already seen how in the area of self-care he did little for himself. On seeing more of the family a picture soon emerged of overprotection and overinvolvement with his mother and elder sister. This was evident in the way the household was organized, who took the decisions and the kinds of feelings expressed by mother towards John. Father said little, but when he did speak he tended to be very emphatic, making his point in an uncompromising, even angry way. He was perceived by the family, particularly by John, as a rather remote and mysterious man. John was a bit frightened of him and thought that he might be capable of being violent. The family was also a relatively 'closed' one, having little contact with outsiders and it was therefore upset by the departure of John's sister who had emigrated to Australia some four years before. This coincided with the worsening in John's work record. In terms of social supports, John had few friends outside the family and no clubs, hobbies or other activities that would take him outside the home. Since he was someone for whom social contacts and activities were likely to be helpful he was given a careful interview to try and build up a picture of what social 'network' he did have and the areas in which this might be improved.

All this information provides the basis for a formulation of the patient's difficulties and the construction of an individualized management plan. The process of assessment is therefore not a simple 'one-off' administration of a test or interview; it can take weeks, even months, to collect all the relevant information and any assessment or formulation is bound to be provisional and reflect only the current state of knowledge about the patient. It may change over time as the outcomes of further investigations and interventions become available. With John it was possible to make a provisional assessment after three to four weeks. This suggested that the reasons for John's failure to maintain stable employment were not due to intellectual deficits, or primarily to task performance problems, but they seemed to be mainly social and motivational. Although it was demonstrated to him that he possessed adequate social skills, for some reason he was unable, or unwilling, to use them. It was hypothesized that he had adopted this childish way of relating to others as a result of differential reinforcement by his mother and elder sister. This was further reinforced by the fact that it enabled him to avoid meeting many of the expectations of independent, adult behaviour, something which he obviously lacked confidence in doing. It was even partially successful in getting people to like him, at least initially. Of course, it was only sucessful in the short-term and there was a price to pay. People soon lost patience with him and it prevented him from any opportunity for constructive, self-expression, i.e. asserting his own wishes, needs and aims. He was unhappy with himself but took some satisfaction in displacing this frustration on to others. In this sense could be described as 'passively aggressive'. As indicated, family factors were seen to play an important role in the aetiology and maintenance of his problem and his functioning seemed to have deteriorated since his sister's departure. Perhaps his sister played a mediating role; they were certainly close and she seems to have been supportive. Father remained a distant, fearful figure and a poor role model for the expression of feelings.

There is much speculation in this kind of formulation and one may wish to disagree with all, or parts, of it. But its function is to bring together the information that we have about John and to give a plausible account of his difficulties. Furthermore, it directs attention to specific aspects of his functioning where interventions might be attempted. This is the next stage in the process.

His basic involvement with the services was good. There were no problems with his physical health and little in the way of psychiatric symptoms. In other cases the assessment might lead to attempts to treat symptoms either by pharmacological or psychological means. As indicated earlier, observations from the whole team of behaviour across a range of settings are important in evaluating such interventions. In the area of self-care the problems have been described: some deficits in skills, but mainly deficits in motivation. Skills can be improved by what is now a fairly standard 'skills training' or 'social learning' approach. This approach employs basic psychological learning theory to improve specific target behaviours. The target is first identified and detailed measures are taken of baseline performance, e.g. daily ratings of personal hygiene or appearance; ratings across a number of specific items concerned with cooking a meal; etc. There are no fixed rules as to what constitutes an adequate baseline, but it must be stable enough such that subsequent progress can be reliably judged. Next, the new target or skill is described. This may involve simple verbal instructions or the therapist may actually need to 'model' (i.e. demonstrate) the new response. When the patient fully understands what he/she is being required to do, they are then asked to practise the new response, e.g. 'now tomorrow please try to remember to comb your hair properly/brush your teeth/not cover your jacket with cigarette-ash', etc. After practising they are given feedback or reinforcement. This is usually in the form of simple praise and encouragement, although sometimes tangible reinforcers (tokens, etc.) may be used. After the reinforcement the next step is to practise again, and again, and again, until a succession of correct responses is achieved.

There are a number of basic points which should always be borne in mind when carrying out this kind of procedure. (1) If 'modelling' is used always direct the patient' attention to that aspect of the model's behaviour that you want him or her to notice (otherwise they won't). (2) Always set the level of a new response at just above the baseline performance; then use the principle of 'shaping' by gradual approximation towards the desired response. This minimizes the danger of arranging yet another failure situation. (3) Reinforce with praise, don't punish. Punishment is rarely effective and one is much better to try to build on the positive. (4) Try to reinforce or give feedback as immediately and as continuously as possible, especially during the acquisition phase. Once established, a new response can be successfully maintained on a more 'partial' schedule of reinforcement. (5) Always use 'over-learning', i.e. repeated practice beyond the first correct production of the response.

It should also be remembered that the arguments for direct, 'in vivo' assessment apply just as well as in the treatment phase. Most psychological treatments have problems with 'generalizing' improvements, i.e. in helping the patient to transfer the gains from an artificial treatment setting to everyday life. If the treatment can also take place as far as possible 'in vivo', these problems of generalization can be reduced. For example, the treatment of social and self-care problems should be carried out in the patient's home and in their local community as much as possible.

Motivational problems are obviously much more difficult to 'treat', but again it depends on an understanding of just what the problem is. In John's case one aspect of the problem was that he seemed to lack confidence in his skills. This was put to him and it was suggested that the only way to improve his confidence was for him to practise those skills and prove to himself that he really could look after himself quite adequately. Another aspect of his motivational problem concerned his parents' attitudes. This was discussed with them and the extent to which they could encourage him to do more and take more responsibility at home was explored. Finally, he was given individual sessions to discuss his general frustrations and his ambivalence about 'growing up'. Motivation' *is* a difficult area, but a good assessment, and sympathetic counselling, can least give you an understanding of what the problem is, even if you are not always successful in eradicating it.

This discussion of skills and motivational problems also applies to the area of work difficulties. John's problems at work were again mainly social and so an individual programme was therefore constructed with the aim of decreasing his childish behaviour at work and increasing appropriate social interactions. This used individual sessions of modelling, role-play and feedback which were than generalized to the actual work settings involving other staff, even other patients, in the reinforcement of appropriate behaviour. John's behaviour was observed and rated every day and he was given bi-weekly feedback on his progress. At the same time some of his problems with social motivation were also discussed. As for the family situation, the assessment and formulation again suggested a number of goals for treatment. John was encouraged to develop positive 'problem-solving' skills at home. He began to learn how to put his point of view across and to express his needs to his parents. They began to learn how to accept them. Mother needed support in order that she might be less over-involved and over-protective. Father also needed encouragement to express his needs more openly and to try to dispel this image of him as a remote, mysterious, possibly dangerous figure. A range of different techniques are useful when working with families depending on the nature of the problem. Family therapy is a difficult area, but progress is possible if we can identify *specific* processes and apply *specific* interventions to them. The final area to consider for treatment is that of social supports. It is obviously not possible to increase someone's range of social activities unless one knows not only what their needs are, but also what facilities are available in their local community. Local information is therefore crucial and the rehabilitation service must be in a position to collect this information and offer it to those who need it. This implies good local knowledge on the part of as many staff as possible and close inter-agency co-operation. The effects of treatment may be evaluated using either single-case methods or with a range of problem-oriented systems of record keeping.

So, we have our assessment and we have tried to treat our patient's problems, however this is by no means the end of the story. In many cases – and John's was one – the patient will not, or cannot, respond to treatment. What do we do then? In the first place, this should not be seen as a failure. Therapy may have failed to produce *improvement* but if we have done it systematically then it should not fail to provide us with *information*. In fact, therapeutic failure is the only way in which chronic disabilities can be defined. How long one should persist in attempts at treatment is difficult to specify; it depends on the patience and the ingenuity of staff, as well as on the provision of resources. Also, the level of chronic disabilities will obviously be different for different individuals and possibly within the same individual for different areas of functioning. Thus, some patients will only be able to cope with a very sheltered living and working environment (e.g. as in a sheltered workshop and supervised hostel); others may require a sheltered work place but be able to manage independent living. We therefore need individualized 'packages' of care and this underlines the need for a wide as possible range of services geared at different levels in each different area of functioning. The long-term management of chronic disabilities is concerned with providing different kinds of environments, tailored to meet these specific needs, which will maintain functioning without necessarily expecting to improve it. The process is therefore: (1) try to help the person change, and (2) if this is not successful, then change the environment and provide whatever degree of shelter is necessary for them to adapt, in spite of their disabilities. The aim is to achieve this while only removing the person minimally from the everyday world.

John was not psychiatrically 'ill' in the usual sense, however his disabilities did prove very difficult to 'treat'. Systematic evaluation of his progress over a period of months suggested that he achieved only small improvements in his abilities to interact more appropriately with others in the work situation and to be more independent and assertive at home. His conflict and ambivalence about 'growing up' remained. He was eventually placed in a sheltered workshop and his parents reluctantly accepted that, for the moment, open employment was not a feasible goal for him. While he remained at home it did not seem likely that any further major changes would occur and at that time neither he, nor they, would consider him leaving home. Contact with the family was maintained with the aim that whatever small gains had been made should not disappear. John is to be reassessed at some time in the future.

To summarize the main points:

1. *The process of rehabilitation can be thought to consist of three basic stages: Assessment, Treatment and Management.*

2. *For assessment purposes the most accurate methods are those based on the direct observation of criterion behaviour.* Formal tests and interviews are of limited value. If direct observation is not possible then useful information may be obtained from a carefully taken history.

3. *Assessment and treatment should be carried out as far as possible in the setting where the problem occurs, or some approximation to it.* The principle of working 'in vivo' is necessary to improve the validity of assessments and to minimize problems of generalizing treatment effects.

4. *Assessment is a gradual accumulation of information about a patient not a single administration of a test.* It is seldom possible to predict *a priori* what level of functioning an individual is likely to achieve in a particular

area. This can only be determined pragmatically, by trying the patient out in various settings and then carefully assessing the outcome.

5. *'Evaluation' in this sense is no different from treatment, they are both part of the procedure of assessing the limits of change.* Evaluation tells one whether or not the intervention has been successful in treating the 'symptom', but whatever the outcome the information that is obtained will still be useful in planning new interventions, or in planning strategies for the management of chronic disabilities. Assessment and treatment are thus linked as two aspects of the same process, i.e. that of defining chronic disabilities.

6. *There are limitations to the treatment model, but just because treatment fails that does not mean that one should necessarily give up.* Successful treatment may be limited for a whole variety of reasons e.g. motivational problems, such as denial or 'secondary gain'; the intransigent attitude of key relatives; the influence of life-events, such as unemployment or bereavement; the unavailability of appropriate resources, etc. Because treatment 'fails' this does not mean that the individual does not require help to manage his disabilities in the long-term. The provision of suitable environments which will maintain functioning in specific areas (work, self-care, social) is as important in rehabilitation as is assessing and improving functioning. This is the true legacy of trying to provide a community-based alternative to the mental hospital.

7. *Rehabilitation must be based on individualized 'packages' of care, not on block treatment or a 'throughput' model.* Individuals are different, both from one another and within their own particular pattern of needs and abilities. Rehabilitation services must recognize these differences and create individualized programmes which contrast with the 'block treatments' of the institutional approach. This is not the 'ladder' model, but rather a process of promoting differential adaptation.

8. *Conclusions in rehabilitation will always be provisional and open to change.* The rehabilitation of the individual has been depicted here as an unfolding process. The conclusions reached in the assessment, or in relation to decisions as to which kind of sheltered environment might be suitable, are determined by the outcomes of the various investigations and interventions. These conclusions will also be affected by subsequent changes in individuals' circumstances. We are all susceptible to life-events and they can have beneficial as well as adverse effects. For example, the death of a parent may remove a long-term disabling motivational block as well as being the cause of an immediate upset.

In summary, planning the rehabilitation of the individual is a time-consuming, difficult and often frustrating exercise. It requires services which are sensitive to the practical demands of everyday life and it also requires organizations which can meet the needs of individuals. Perhaps, above all it requires staff who can accept their limitations. There is nothing wrong with trying to 'treat' people, just as long as failure is met with the same enthusiasm and optimism as success. Rehabilitation is often as much about 'failure' as it is about success and the pressures to then fall back on institutional practices are always great. These pressures can only be resisted by staff who know what they are doing, why they are doing it, and who are sufficiently self-critical and open that they can change how they are working if needs demand.

# References

Allderidge, P. (1979) Hospitals, madhouses and asylums: cycles in the care of the insane, *British Journal of Psychiatry*, **134**, 321–34.

Bachrach, L. L. (1976) *Deinstitutionalization: an analytical review and sociological perspective*, US Department of Health, Education, and Welfare: Maryland.

Bachrach, L. L. (1978) A conceptual approach to deinstitutionalization, *Hospital and Community Psychiatry*, **29**, 573–8.

Baker, R., Hall, J. N. and Hutchinson, K. (1974) A token economy project with chronic schizophrenic patients, *British Journal of Psychiatry*, **124**, 367–84.

Baker, R., Hall, J. N., Hutchinson, K., and Bridge, G. (1977) Symptom changes in chronic schizophrenic patients in a token economy: a controlled experiment, *British Journal of Psychiatry*, **131**, 381–93.

Balla, D. A. (1976) Relationship of institution size to quality of care: a review of the literature, *American Journal of Mental Deficiency*, **81**, 117–24.

Beck, A. T., Rush, A. J., Shaw, B. F., and Emery, G. (1979) *Cognitive therapy of depression*, Guildford Press: New York.

Beels, C. C. (1981) Social support and schizophrenia, *Schizophrenia Bulletin*, **7(1)**, 58–72.

Bender, M. (1979) Community psychology: when?, *Bulletin of the British Psychological Society*, **32**, 6–9.

Bennett, D. H. (1970) the value of work in psychiatric rehabilitation, *Social Psychiatry*, **4**, 224–30.

Bennett, D. H. (1973) Community mental health services in Britain, *American Journal of Psychiatry*, **130**, 1065–70.

Bennett, D. H. (1976a) Day Treatment in England, Paper given at Multi-Disciplinary National Forum on Adult Psychiatric Day Treatment, University of Minneapolis: Minnesota.

Bennett, D. H. (1976b) Techniques of industrial therapy, ergotherapy and recreative methods in K. P. Kisker, J. E. Meiper, C. Müler and E. Strömgren (eds), *Psychiatric der Gegenwart*, Vol. III, Springer: Berlin.

Bennett, D. H. (1978a) Social forms of psychiatric treatment, in J. K. Wing (ed.) *Schizophrenia: Towards a New Synthesis*, Academic Press: London.

Bennett, D. H. (1978b) The role of the day hospital, in *Report of a Seminar on Day Care for the Mentally Ill*, DHSS: London.

Bennett, D. H. (1978c) The Camberwell district psychiatric services 1964–1974: the provision of alternatives to mental hospital care, in L. I. Stein and M. A. Test (eds), *Alternatives to Mental Hospital Treatment*, Plenum Press: New York.

Bennett, D. H. (1980) The chronic psychiatric patient today, *Journal of the Royal Society of Medicine*, **73**, 301–3.

Bennett, D. H. (1981a) Psychiatric day services: a cornerstone of care, in *New Directions for Psychiatric Day Services*, MIND: London.

Bennett, D. H. (1981b) The Camberwell district rehabilitation service, in J. K. Wing and B. Morris (eds). *Handbook of Psychiatric Rehabilitation Practice*, Oxford University Press: Oxford.

Bennett, D., Fox, C., Jowell, T. and Skynner, A. C. R. (1976) Towards a family approach in a psychiatric day hospital, *Britain Journal of Psychiatry*, **129**, 73–81.

Birley, J. L. T. (1974) A housing association for psychiatric patients, *Psychiatric Quarterly*, **48**, 568–71.

Bockoven, J. S. (1963) *Moral treatment in psychiatry*, Springer Publications: New York.

Brandon, D. (1981) MIND (The National Association for Mental Health), in J. K. Wing and B. Morris (eds), *Handbook of Psychiatric Rehabilitation Practice*, Oxford University Press: Oxford.

Brehm, S. (1976) *The application of social psychology to clinical practice*, Hemisphere Books: New York.

Brown, G. W. (1959) Experiences of discharged chronic schizophrenic mental hospital patients in various types of living group, *Millbank Memorial Fund Quarterly*, **37**, 105–34.

Brown, G. W. and Birley, J. L. T. (1968) Crises and life changes and the onset of schizophrenia, *Journal of Health and Social Behaviour*, **9**, 203–14.

Brown, G. W., Birley, J. L. T. and Wing, J. K. (1972) Influence of family life on the course of schizophrenic disorders: a replication, *British Journal of Psychiatry*, **121**, 241–58.

Brown, G. W., Bone, M., Dalison, M. and Wing, J. K. (1966) *Schizophrenia and social care*, Oxford University Press: Oxford.

Brown, G. W. and Harris, T. (1978) *Social origins of depression*, Tavistock: London.

Brown, G. W., Monck, G. M., Carstairs, G. and Wing, J. K. (1962) Influence of family life on the course of schizophrenic illness, *British Journal of Preventative and Social Medicine*, **16**, 55–68.

Caplan, G. (1964) *Principles of preventive psychiatry*, Basic Books: New York.

Christie-Brown, J. R. W., Ebringer, L. and Freedman, K. S. (1977) A survey of long-stay psychiatric population: implications for community services, *Psychological Medicine*, **7**, 113–26.

Clark, D. (1974) *Social therapy in psychiatry*, Penguin Books: Harmondsworth.

Cochrane, A. (1971) *Effectiveness and efficiency – random reflections on health services*, Oxford University Press: Oxford.

Collins, J., Kreitman, W., Nelson, B., and Troop, J. (1971) Neurosis and marital interaction. III: family roles and functions, *British Journal of Psychiatry*, **119**, 233–42.

Cook, T. D. and Campbell, D. T. (1979) *Quasi-experimentation – design to analysis issues for field settings*, Rand McNally: Chicago.

Cooper, B. (1966) Psychiatric disorder in Hospital and general practice, *Social Psychiatry*, **1**, 7–10.

Cooper, J. and Sartorius, N. (1977) Cultural and temporal variations in schizophrenia: a speculation on the importance of industrialization, *British Journal of Psychiatry*, **130**, 50–5.

Crossman, R. (1979) *The diaries of a Cabinet Minister*, A. Howard (ed.), Magnum Books: London.

Davis, A. E., Dintz, S. and Pasamanick, B. (1972) The prevention of hospitalization in schizophrenia: five years after an experimental program, *American Journal of Orthopsychiatry*, **42**, 375–88.

Department of Health and Social Security (1975) Personal social services: local authority statistics, adult day centres 1973–1975, HMSO: London.

Department of Health and Social Security (1979) Organizational and management problems of mental illness hospitals – report of a working group, DHSS: London.

Dohrenwend, B. P. and Dohrenwend, B. S. (1974) Social and cultural influences on psychopathology, *Annual Review of Psychology*, **25**, 417–52.

Duncan-Jones, P., (1981) The structure of social relationships: analysis of a survey instrument, *Social Psychiatry*, **16**, 55–61.

Dunham, H. W. (1976) Society, culture and mental disorder, *Archives of General Psychiatry*, **33**, 147–57.

Ebringer, L. and Christie-Brown, J. R. W. (1980) Social deprivation amongst short stay psychiatric patients, *British Journal of Psychiatry*, **136**, 46–52.

Edwards, C. (1981) Research looks at practice difficulties, in *New Directions for Psychiatric Day Services*, MIND: London.

Edwards, C. and Carter, J. (1979) Day services and the mentally ill, in J. K. Wing and R. Olsen (eds), *Community Care for the Mentally Disabled*, Oxford University Press: Oxford.

Eisenberg, P. and Lazarsfeld, P. F. (1938) The psychological effects of unemployment, *Psychological Bulletin*, **35**, 358–90.

Ekdawi, M. K. (1981) Counselling in Rehabilitation, in J. K. Wing and B. Morris (eds), *Handbook of Psychiatric Rehabilitation Practice*, Oxford University Press: Oxford.

Elliot, P. A., Barlow, F., Hooper, A. and Kingerlee, P. E. (1979) Maintaining patients' improvements in a token economy, *Behaviour Research and Therapy*, **17**, 355–67.

Ellsworth, R. B., Collins, J. F., Casey, N. A., Schoonover, R. A., Hickey, R. H., Hyer, L.,Twemlow, S. W., Nesselroade, J. R. (1979) Some characteristics of effective psychiatric treatment programs, *Journal of Consulting and Clinical Psychology*, **47**, 799–817.

Erickson, R. C. (1975) Outcome studies in mental hospitals: a review, *Psychological Bulletin*, **82**, 519–40.

Fairweather, G. W., Sanders, D. H. and Tornatsky, L. G.

(1974) *Creating change in mental health organisations*, Pergamon Press: New York.

Falloon, I. R. H., Liberman, R. P., Lillie, F. J. and Vaughn, C. (1981) Family therapy of schizophrenics with high risk relapse, *Family Process*, **20**, 211–21.

Fenton, F. R., Tessier, L., Struening, E. L., Smith, F. A. and Bendit, C. (1982) *Home and hospital psychiatric treatment*, Croom Helm: London.

Fontana, A. F. and Dowds, B. N. (1975) Assessing treatment outcome I. Adjustment in the community, *Journal of Nervous and Mental Diseases*, **161**, 221–30.

Foot, M. (1975) *Aneurin Bevan*, Vol. 2, 1945–1960, Paladin Books: London.

Georgiades, N. J. and Phillimore, L. (1975) The myth of the hero-innovator and alternative strategies for organisational change, in C. C. Kiernan and F. D. Woodford (eds), *Behaviour Modification with the Severely Retarded*, Associated Scientific Publishers: Amsterdam.

Glick, I. D. and Hargreaves, W. A. (1979) *Psychiatric hospital treatment for the 1980s*, Lexington Books: Lexington, Mass.

Glick, I. D. and Kessler, D. R. (1980) *Marital and family therapy*, Grune and Stratton: New York.

Goffman, E. (1961) *Asylums: essays on the social situation of mental patients and other inmates*, Anchor Books, Doubleday: New York.

Goldberg, D. and Blackwell, B. (1970) Psychiatric illness in general practice. A detailed study using a new method of case identification, *British Medical Journal*, **2**, 439–43.

Goldberg, D. and Huxley, P. (1980) *Mental illness in the community*, Tavistock Publications: London.

Gruenberg, E. M. (1967) The social-breakdown syndrome – some origins, *American Journal of Psychiatry*, **123**, 12–20.

Gunderson, J. G. (1980) A re-evaluation of milieu therapy for non-chronic schizophrenic patients, *Schizophrenic Bulletin*, **6**, 64–9.

Gunn, J. (1977) Criminal behaviour and mental disorder, *British Journal of Psychiatry*, **130**, 317–29.

Hall, J. N. and Baker, R. D. (1972) Practical Difficulties in the Implementation of Token Economy Programmes, Paper presented at the Second European Conference on Behaviour

Modification, Wexford: Ireland.

Hall, J. N., Baker, R. D., and Hutchison, K. (1977) A controlled evaluation of token economy procedures with chronic schizophrenic patients. *Behaviour Research and Therapy*, **15**, 261–83.

Hartley, J. (1980) Psychological approaches to unemployment, *Bulletin of the British Psychological Society*, **32**, 309–14.

Hawks, D. V. (1971) Can clinical psychology afford to treat the individual?, *Bulletin of the British Psychological Society*, **24**, 133–5.

Heller, K. (1979) Social support, chapter in A. P. Goldstein and F. H. Kander (eds), *Maximising Treatment Gains*, Academic Press: New York.

Henderson, S. (1977) The social network, support and neurosis. The function of attachment in adult life, *British Journal of Psychiatry*, **131**, 185–91.

Henderson, S. (1980) A development in social psychiatry: the systematic study of social bonds, *Journal of Nervous and Mental Diseases*, **168**, 63–9.

Henderson, S., Duncan-Jones, P., McAuley, H. and Ritchie, K. (1978a) The patients' primary group, *British Journal of Psychiatry*, **132**, 74–86.

Henderson, S., Byrne, D. G., Duncan-Jones, P., Adcock, S., Scott, R. and Steele, G. P. (1978b) Social bonds in the epidemiology of neurosis: a preliminary communication, *British Journal of Psychiatry*, **132**, 463–6.

Henderson, S., Duncan-Jones, P., Byrne, D. G. and Scott, R. (1980a) Measuring social relationships – the interview schedule for social interaction, *Psychological Medicine*, **10**, 723–34.

Henderson, S., Byrne, D. G., Duncan-Jones, P., Scott, R. and Adcock, S. (1980b) Social relationships, adversity and neurosis: a study of association in a general population sample, *British Journal of Psychiatry*, **136**, 574–83.

Herz, M. I., Endicott, J. and Spitzer, R. L. (1975) Brief hospitalization of patients with families: Initial results, *American Journal of Psychiatry*, **132**, 413–18.

Herz, M. I., Endicott, J. and Spitzer, R. L. (1976) Brief versus standard hospitalization: the families, *American Journal of Psychiatry*, **133**, 795–801.

Herz, M. I., Endicott, J. and Spitzer, R. L. (1977) Brief hospitalization: a two year follow-up, *American Journal of Psychiatry*, **134**, 502–7.

Herz, M. I., Endicott, J., Spitzer, R. L. and Mesnikoff, A. (1971) Day versus in-patient hospitalization: a controlled study, *American Journal of Psychiatry*, **127**, 107–18.

Hewett, S. H., Ryan, P. and Wing, J. K. (1975) Living without the mental hospitals, *Journal of Social Policy*, **4**, 391–404.

Horwitz, A. (1977) The pathways into psychiatric treatment: some differences between men and women, *Journal of Health and Social Behaviour*, **18**.

Ingleby, D. (1981) Understanding mental illness, in D. Ingleby (ed.), *Critical Psychiatry*, Penguin Books: Harmondsworth.

Jablensky, A. and Sartorius, N. (1975) Culture and schizophrenia, *Psychological Medicine*, **5**, 113–24.

Jacob, T. (1975) Family interaction in disturbed and normal families: a methodological and substantive review, *Psychological Bulletin*, **82**, 33–65.

Jacques, E. (1967) *Equitable payment*, Penguin Books: Harmondsworth.

Jahoda, M. (1979) The impact of unemployment in the 1930s and the 1970s, *Bulletin of the British Psychological Society*, **32**, 309–14.

Jones, K. (1972) *A history of the mental health services*, Routledge & Kegan Paul: London.

Jones, M. (1968) *Beyond the therapeutic community: social learning and social psychiatry*, Yale University Press: Newhaven, Connecticut.

Jones-Parry, W. (1972) *The trade in lunacy*, Routledge & Kegan Paul: London.

Jowell, T. (1981) The Brecknock community and mental health project, in *New Directions for Psychiatric Day Services*, MIND: London.

Kanfer, F. (1979) Self-management: strategies and tactics, chapter in A. P. Goldstein and F. H. Kanfer (eds), *Maximising Treatment Gains*, Academic Press: New York.

Keddie, A. C. (1978) The Influence of Dayroom Seating Arrangement on Behaviour in a Psychiatric Hospital Ward, MSc. Thesis, University of Exeter (unpublished).

King, R., Raynes, N. and Tizard, J. (1971) *Patterns of residential care*, Routledge & Kegan Paul: London.

Kogan, N. and Wallach, M. A. (1967) Risk taking as a function of the situation, the person, and the group, *New Directions in Psychology*, Vol. 3, Holt Rhinehart and Winston: New York.

Kuipers, L. (1979) Schizophrenia and the family. Part I: the problems of relatives, in J. K. Wing and R. Olsen (eds), *Community Care for the Mentally Disabled*, Oxford University Press: Oxford.

Lamb, R. H. (1979) The new asylums in the community, *Archives of General Psychiatry*, **36**, 129–34.

Leach, J. (1979) Providing for the destitute, in J. K. Wing and R. Olsen (eds), *Community Care for the Mentally Disabled*, Oxford University Press: Oxford.

Leach, J. and Wing, J. (1980) *Helping destitute men*, Tavistock Publications: London.

Leff, J. P. (1978) Social and psychological causes of the acute attack, in J. K. Wing (ed.), *Schizophrenia: Towards a New Synthesis*, Academic Press: London.

Lewis, S. (1981) The care of severely disabled long-stay patients, in J. K. Wing and B. Morris (eds), *Handbook of Psychiatric Rehabilitation Practice*, Oxford University Press: Oxford.

Liem, R. and Liem, J. (1978) Social class and mental illness reconsidered: the role of economic stress and social support, *Journal of Health and Social Behaviour*, **19**, 139–56.

Litman, G. K., Eiser, J. R., Rawson, N. S. B., Oppenheim, A. N. (1979) Differences in relapse precipitants and coping behaviour between alcohol relapsers and survivors, *Behaviour Research and Therapy*, **17**, 89–94.

Lomax, M. (1921) *The experiences of an asylum doctor*, George Allen & Unwin: London.

McMiller, P. and Ingham, J. G. (1976) Friends, confidants and symptoms, *Social Psychiatry*, **11**, 51–8.

McPeak, W. R. (1979) Family therapies, in A. P. Goldstein and F. H. Kanfer (eds), *Maximising Treatment Gains*, Academic Press: New York.

Mann, S. A. and Cree, W. (1976) 'New' long-stay psychiatric patients: a national sample survey of fifteen mental hospitals in England and Wales 1972/3, *Psychological Medicine*, **6**, 603–16.

Martin, S. (1981) Lessons from the experience of a day centre in the Worcester development project, in *New directions for psychiatric day services*, MIND: London.

Meichenbaum, D. (1977) *Cognitive-behaviour modification*: *an integrative approach*, Plenum Press: New York.

Menzies, I. E. P. (1970) *The functioning of social systems as a defence against anxiety*, Tavistock pamphlet No. 3,: London.

Miles, A. (1971) Long-stay schizophrenic patients in hospital workshops: a comparative study of an industrial unit and an occupational therapy department, *British Journal of Psychiatry*, **119**, 611–22.

Miles, A. (1972) The development of interpersonal relationships among long-stay patients in two hospital workshops, *British Journal of Medical Psychology*, **45**, 105–14.

Miles, A. (1981) *The mentally ill in contemporary society: a sociological introduction*, Martin Robertson: Oxford.

Miller, E. J. and Gwynne, G. V. (1972) *A life apart*, Tavistock Publications: London.

MIND (1961) *Report of the annual conference*, MIND: London.

MIND (1980) *Mental health statistics*, MIND: London.

Mischel, W. (1968) *Personality and assessment*, Wileys: New York.

Morris, B. (1981) Residential units, in J. K. Wing and B. Morris (eds) *Handbook of Psychiatric Rehabilitation Practice*, Oxford University Press: Oxford.

Murray, J. (1978) Special housing. MIND: London.


Neale, J. M. and Oltmanns, T. F. (1980) *Schizophrenia* Wileys: New York.


Paul, G. (1969) The chronic mental patient: current status – future directions, *Psychological Bulletin*, **71**, 81–94.

Paul, G. L. and Lentz, R. J. (1977) *Psychosocial treatment of chronic mental patients: milieu vs. social-learning programs*, Harvard University Press: Harvard, Mass.

Pearlin, L. I. and Schooler, C. (1978) The structure of coping, *Journal of Health and Social Behaviour*, **19**, 2–21.

Priestley, D. (1979) Schizophrenia and the family part II. Helping a self-help group, in J. K. Wing and R. Olsen (eds), *Community Care for the Mentally Disabled*, Oxford University Press: Oxford.


Raynes, N. V., Pratt, M. W. and Roses, S. (1974) *Final report: organisational structure and care in institutions for the retarded*,

US Department of Health Education and Welfare, Grant HD 04147 Mimeo: Mass.

Raynes, N., Pratt, M. and Roses, S. (1979) *Organizational structure and the Care of the mentally handicapped*, Croom Helm: London.

Rezin, V. A., Elliot, P. A. and Paschalis, P. (1979) Nurse-patient Interaction in a Token Economy, Paper presented at the Annual Conference of the British Association for Behavioural Psychotherapy, Bangor: North Wales.

Rothman, D. J. (1971) *The discovery of the asylum*, Little Brown & Company: Boston.

Rutter, M., Maughan, B., Mortimore, P., Ouston, J. and Smith, A. (1979) *Fifteen thousand hours: secondary schools and their effects on children*, Open Books: London.

Ryan, P. (1979) Residential care for the mentally disabled, in J. K. Wing and R. Olsen (eds), *Community Care for the Mentally Disabled*, Oxford University Press: Oxford.

Ryan, P. and Hewett, S. H. (1976) A pilot study of hostels for the mentally ill, *Social Work Today*, **6**, 774–8.

Sanson-Fisher, R. W., Poole, A. D. and Thompson, V. (1979) Behaviour patterns within a general hospital psychiatric unit: an observational study, *Behaviour Research and Therapy*, **17**, 317–32.

Sartorius, N., Jablensky, A. and Shapiro, R. (1977) Two-year follow-up of the patients included in the WHO international pilot study of schizophrenia, *Psychological Medicine*, **7**, 529–41.

Schumacher, E. F. (1973) *Small is beautiful – A study of economics as if people mattered*, Blond Briggs: London.

Secord, P. F. and Backman, C. W. (1964) *Social psychology*, McGraw Hill: New York.

Shepherd, G. (1977) Social skills training: the generalisation problem, *Behaviour Therapy*, **8**, 1008–9.

Shepherd, G. (1978) Social skills training; The generalisation problem – some further data, *Behaviour Research and Therapy*, **16**, 287–8.

Shepherd, G. (1980) The treatment of social difficulties in special environments, in M. P. Feldman and J. Orford (eds) *Psychological Problems: The Social Context*, Wileys: Chichester.

Shepherd, G. (1981a) Day care and the chronic patient, in *New directions for psychiatric day services*, MIND: London.

Shepherd, G. (1981b) Psychological disorder and unemployment, *Bulletin of the British Psychological Society*, **34**, 345–8.

Shepherd, G. (1982) A Survey of Potential Long-term Patients Currently Resident on Acute Admission Wards, Department of Psychology, Fulbourn Hospital: Cambridge (unpublished).

Shepherd, G. (1983a) Planning the rehabilitation of the individual, in F. N. Watts and D. H. Bennett (eds), *Theory and Practice in Psychiatric Rehabilitation*, Wileys: Chichester.

Shepherd, G. (1983b) Introduction, in S. Spence and G. Shepherd (eds), *Developments in Social Skills Training*, Academic Press: London.

Shepherd, G. and Richardson, A. (1979a) Organisation and interaction in psychiatric day centres, *Psychological Medicine*, **9**, 573–9.

Shepherd, G. and Richardson, A. (1979b) Social skills and beyond: environments for the care of chronic problems, *Behavioural Psychotherapy*, **7**, 31–8.

Sinclair, I. (1975) The influence of wardens and matrons of probation hostels, in J. Tizard, I. Sinclair, R. V. G. Clarke (eds), *Varieties of Residential Experience*, Routledge and Kegan Paul: London.

Stein, L. I. and Test, M. A. (1978) An alternative to mental hospital treatment, in L. I. Stein and M. A. Test (eds), *Alternatives to Mental Hospital Treatment*, Plenum Press: New York.

Stokes, G. (1982) The Meaning of Work and the Personal Cost of unemployment, Paper presented at West Midlands Division of Clinical Psychology Symposium of Psychological Aspects of Unemployment, Birmingham, February (unpublished).

Strauss, J. S. and Carpenter, W. T. (1974) The prediction of outcome in schizophrenia II. Relationships between predictor and outcome variables, *Archives of General Psychiatry*, **31**, 37–42.

Sutton, G. (1981) The organisation and administration of nursing services for long-stay patients, in J. K. Wing and B. Morris (eds), *Handbook of Psychiatric Rehabilitation Practice*, Oxford University Press: Oxford.

Test, M. A. and Stein L. I. (1978) Training in community living: research design and results, in L. I. Stein and M. A. Test (eds), *Alternatives to Mental Hospital Treatment*, Plenum Press: New York.

Tharp, R. G. and Wetzel, R. J. (1969) *Behaviour modification in the natural environment*, Academic Press: New York.

Townsend, J. M. (1976) Self-concept and the institutionalization of mental patients: an overview and critique, *Journal of Health and Social Behaviour*, **17**, 263–71.

Treacher, A. and Baruch, G. (1981) Towards a critical history of the psychiatric profession, in D. Ingleby (ed.), *Critical Psychiatry*, Penguin Books: Harmondsworth.

Truax, C. B. and Carkhuff, R. R. (1967) *Toward effective counseling and psychotherapy*, Aldine: Chicago.

Vaughn, C. E. and Leff, J. P. (1976) The influence of family and social factors on the course of psychiatric illness, *British Journal of Psychiatry*, **129**, 125–38.

Walrond-Skinner, S. (1981) *Developments in family therapy: theories and applications since 1948*, Routledge & Kegan Paul: London.

Wansborough, S. N. (1981) The place of work in rehabilitation, in J. K. Wing and B. Morris (eds), *Handbook of Psychiatric Rehabilitation Practice*, Oxford University Press: Oxford.

Wansbrough, N. and Cooper, P. (1980) *Open employment after mental illness*, Tavistock Publications: London.

Watts, F. N. (1978) A study of work behaviour in a psychiatric rehabilitation unit, *British Journal of Social and Clinical Psychology*, **17**, 85–92.

Watts, F. N. and Bennett, D. H. (1977) Previous occupational stability as a predictor of employment after psychiatric rehabilitation, *Psychological Medicine*, **7**, 709–12.

Watts, F. N. and Bennett, D. H. (1983) Management of the staff team, in F. N. Watts and D. H. Bennett (eds), *Theory and Practice in Psychiatric Rehabilitation*, Wileys: Chichester.

Weisbrod, B. A., Test, M. A. and Stein, L. I. (1980) Alternatives to mental hospital treatment II. Economic cost-benefit analysis, *Archives of General Psychiatry*, **37**, 400–5.

Weiss, R. S. (1974) The provision of social relationships, in Z. Rubin (ed.), *Doing Unto Others*, Prentice Hall: New York.

Whatmore, R., Durward, L. and Kushlick, A. (1975) Measuring the quality of residential care, *Behaviour Research and Therapy*, **13**, 227–36.

Wilder, J. (1981) The Psychiatric Rehabilitation Association, in J. K. Wing and B. Morris (eds), *Handbook of Psychiatric Rehabilitation Practice*, Oxford University Press: Oxford.

Wing, J. K. (1978a) Clinical concepts of schizophrenia, in J. K. Wing (ed.) *Schizophrenia: Towards a New Synthesis*, Academic Press: London.

Wing, J. K. (1978b) Who becomes chronic?, *Psychiatric Quarterly*, **50**, 178–90.

Wing, J. K. (1978c) Planning and evaluating services for chronically handicapped patients in the United Kingdom, in L. I. Stein and M. A. Test (eds), *Alternatives to Mental Hospital Treatment*, Plenum Press: New York.

Wing, J. K., Bennett, D. H. and Denham, J. (1964) Industrial Rehabilitation of Long-Stay Schizophrenic Patients, Medical Research Council Memo. No. 42, HMSO: London.

Wing, J. K. and Brown, G. W. (1970) *Institutionalism and schizophrenia: a comparative study of three mental hospitals, 1960–1968*, Cambridge University Press: Cambridge.

Wing, J. K. and Creer, C. (1980) Schizophrenia at home, in H. R. Rollin (ed.), *Coping with Schizophrenia*, for National Schizophrenia Fellowship, Burnett Books: London.

Wing, J. K. and Hailey, A. M. (1972) *Evaluating a community psychiatric service: the Camberwell register, 1964–71*, Oxford University Press: Oxford.

Wing, J. K. and Morris, B. (1981) Clinical basis of rehabilitation, in J. K. Wing and B. Morris (eds), *Handbook of Psychiatric Rehabilitation Practice*, Oxford University Press: Oxford.

Wing, J. K. and Olsen, R. (1979) Principles of the new community care, in J. K. Wing and R. Olsen (eds), *Community Care for the Mentally Disabled*, Oxford University Press: Oxford.

Wykes, T. (1982), A hostel-ward for 'new' long-stay patients: an evaluative study of 'A ward in a house', in J. K. Wing (ed.), *Long-term Community, Care: Experience in a London Borough*, Psychological Monograph Supplement 2, Cambridge University Press: Cambridge.

Young, M. and Willmott, P. (1975) *The symmetrical family*, Penguin Books: Harmondsworth.

Zigler, E. and Phillips, L. (1961) Social competence and outcome in psychiatric disorder, *Journal of Abnormal and Social Psychology*, **63**, 264–71.

D'Zurilla, T. J. and Goldfried, M. R. (1971) Problem solving and behaviour modification, *Journal of Abnormal Psychology*, **78**, 107–26.

# Index